Advance Praise for *Lilias! Yoga*

"In this exquisite book, Lilias has deftly communicated both the essence of yoga and the essence of Lilias. The book is so inviting that one just wants to fall into it—and into the warmth and wisdom of Lilias's teaching. This kind of work can only be the fruit of a lifetime of dedicated practice—and we are enormously grateful to have it, and to have Lilias."

—Stephen Cope, director of the Kripalu Institute for Extraordinary Living and author of *Yoga and the Quest for the True Self*

"Lilias Folan simply and profoundly demystifies the higher teachings of yoga and meditation. Highly recommended for students and teachers alike."

—Larry Payne, Ph.D., coauthor of *Yoga for Dummies* and *Yoga R$_x$* and founding president of the International Association of Yoga Therapists

"Whenever I see Lilias, I think, 'I'll have what she's having!' In her new book, Lilias's teachings, which gracefully balance wisdom with play, clearly show us that we *can* experience the strength, joy, and clarity that Lilias herself radiates. Thank you, Lilias!"

—Cyndi Lee, founder of OM yoga

"In this book, Lilias Folan reminds us that authentic spiritual paths are not a function of age, because genuine wisdom is ageless. This includes the great tradition of yoga, of which Folan has done so much to bring to Western awareness. [*Lilias! Yoga*] will help anyone recover the joy and fulfillment of graceful aging."

—Larry Dossey, M.D., author of *The Extraordinary Healing Power of Ordinary Things* and *Healing Words*

"Lilias paved the way for so many of us. She was the first American yoga celebrity—and I mean that in the most complimentary way. Lilias was the pioneer and introduced yoga to America so sweetly. Thank God she was first! With her light and genuine love of people, she gently awakened people's interest in yoga. . . . She has always been an inspiration for me and my work, and now this lovely book from her for all of us growing older—and isn't everyone?"

—Beryl Bender Birch, author of *Power Yoga* and *Beyond Power Yoga*

"The beloved doyenne of American yoga has done it again, offered us a jewel. This new book is both a friendly and deeply spiritual guide to the power of yoga practice through all the stages of our lives. Lilias has lived its wisdom, and now we can share that wisdom, as well as the joy she radiates as she teaches us."

—Judith Hanson Lasater, Ph.D., physical therapist, yoga teacher since 1971, and author of several books, including *30 Essential Poses*

"The luminous Lilias has given us a book as wise as it is essential to the enhancement of the body, mind, and soul of the mature person. Here is yoga for the new millennium as we live longer lives with joy and greater usefulness."

—Jean Houston, Ph.D., codirector of the Foundation for Mind Research in Ashland, Oregon, and author of *A Passion for the Possible*

"People at midlife and beyond—myself included—want to hear from seasoned teachers who have stood the test of time. Lilias has the depth of experience to provide older students with inspiration, encouragement, and practical guidance. She demonstrates how yoga can help us to reconnect with inner peace and joy. I wholeheartedly agree with Lilias that yoga gets better with age!"

—Suza Francina, R.Y.T., author of *The New Yoga for People over 50*

"I have had the privilege of collaborating with Lilias in the development of many of her video projects throughout the years. I have always found the time that we spend together to be sacred. She has shown me through example how to live each day with warmth and serenity."

—Debra Goldman, founder of Natural Journeys

"A gentle, wise path toward understanding, awareness, and health. Heed these instructions and you will get better with age too."

—Barbara Dossey, Ph.D., R.N., author of *Florence Nightingale* and *Holistic Nursing*

"Lilias expresses the wisdom and compassion of a Yogini with a lifetime of expertise. She is an American icon and this book is her gift to the world."

—Jimmy Barkan, founder of Hot Yoga with Jimmy Barkan Studio, Yoga Connection of South Florida

"Lilias's motivation is so obviously one of genuine caring and inspiration that her work has a quality of gentle power and deep meaning. Lilias Folan is one of those rare people who can teach an ancient wisdom and also infuse it with a modern and tender regard for her students. . . this is excellence. I am grateful to have this book."

—Patricia Sun, spiritual teacher and director of the Institute of Communication and Understanding in Berkeley, California

"Lilias yoga has been a longstanding prescription for my patients that has yielded consistently positive results. Lilias reveals an intimate and heartwarming yoga guide that encourages readers to enhance inward and outward health at midlife and beyond. Through her characteristic warmth and creativity, Lilias continues to inspire and awe."

—Kenna Stephenson, M.D., F.A.A.F.P., author of *Awakening Athena*

"Lilias, our grand Diva of American yoga, has blessed us with a book that takes us on a spiritual journey and reveals to us that it *does* get better with age. She brings to the reader her heartfelt approach and experience to all aspects of spiritual practice. . . . Her simple step by step approach to the asanas, pranayama, and meditation invites couples and individuals to make yoga a part of their lives and affirms that it's never too late to do yoga."

—Elise Browning Miller, author of *Yoga: Anytime, Anywhere*

"[*Lilias! Yoga*] offers inspiration and fresh approaches to the practice of yoga—for beginners, long-time students, and teachers alike. It is a treasure map, a reference manual for so much more than a physical practice. Lilias offers a heart-centered approach to yoga that honors the different stages of life."

—Marti Glenn, Ph.D., president of the Santa Barbara Graduate Institute

"This book is brilliant, both enlightening and life enhancing. Lilias's yogic treasures stream from the pages and allow us to experience both the benefits and compassion of true yoga. This is not just a 'look good' yoga book—it is the real thing!"

—Liz Comerton, cofounder and past president of the Yoga Fellowship of Northern Ireland

Lilias! YOGA

YOUR GUIDE TO ENHANCING BODY, MIND, AND SPIRIT IN MIDLIFE AND BEYOND

LILIAS FOLAN

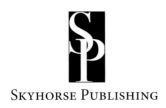

Skyhorse Publishing

Cover photograph courtesy of Naturaljourneys®
www.naturaljourneys.com

Copyright © 2011 by Lilias Folan

All Rights Reserved. No part of this book may be reproduced in any manner without the express written consent of the publisher, except in the case of brief excerpts in critical reviews or articles. All inquiries should be addressed to Skyhorse Publishing, 307 West 36th Street, 11th Floor, New York, NY 10018.

Skyhorse Publishing books may be purchased in bulk at special discounts for sales promotion, corporate gifts, fund-raising, or educational purposes. Special editions can also be created to specifications. For details, contact the Special Sales Department, Skyhorse Publishing, 307 West 36th Street, 11th Floor, New York, NY 10018 or info@skyhorsepublishing.com.

Skyhorse® and Skyhorse Publishing® are registered trademarks of Skyhorse Publishing, Inc.®, a Delaware corporation.

www.skyhorsepublishing.com

10 9 8 7 6 5 4 3 2 1

Library of Congress Cataloging-in-Publication Data is available on file.

ISBN: 978-1-61608-451-6

Printed in China

The instructions for the focused meditation on pages 118–119 are from *Yoga R$_x$* by Larry Payne, Ph.D., and Richard Usatine, M.D. (Broadway Books, 2002: p. 57). Used with permission.

All photographs by Circe Hamilton
Book design by Christina Gaugler

This book is dedicated to my awesome students and my very dear family. You are my teachers. And, like all great teachers, you've taught me lessons I never thought I needed to learn. Thank you for your patience, warm affection, and cheerful support. I carry your light carefully and gratefully in my heart.

Contents

Foreword
Lilias: Everything Gets Better with Age

Over the years I've witnessed a remarkable transformation. I've been fortunate to know Lilias as she has *become* yoga. I'm not speaking about the TV personality, the teacher, the writer, the woman, the daughter, the sister, the mother, the wife, or the friend. I'm talking about the one who is living behind and within all these roles; the one I call a spiritual sister; the one I've had the privilege of knowing for almost 30 years; the one I've traveled and taught with from California to Assisi, Italy. And the one with whom I've shared the joys of this journey of life through its many challenges of raising a family, teaching, and walking this precious path called yoga.

I've seen Lilias transform from being a teacher *of* yoga into being embodied *as* yoga. Lilias isn't practicing or teaching yoga anymore, she's *being* yoga. Lilias has become what yoga preaches; she is meditation in action. It's not that moments of confusion, restlessness, or anxiety have altogether disappeared. Something much deeper has transpired. Lilias has grown into being the amazing secret that yoga reveals. We call it the *Open Secret* because it's available to everyone, yet most of us don't recognize it even when we're experiencing it. It's like a great elephant that's resting quietly in our living room, but for some odd reason, we don't see it. Well, Lilias has!

And what is this secret? Lilias has stopped pretending that she should be someone else. Lilias knows her inner witness that is without judgment, that knows and sees and accepts everything as it is and everyone just as they are. She has arrived at the center of this hurricane called life. Here, life continues, thoughts keep coming, but Lilias knows herself as *stillness*, the inner spiritual essence that we all are, that knows no lack or separation. Here, as Buddha so eloquently said, is the end of suffering. Lilias knows what life is truly about. She is living as the *mystery* from which everything is born and back into which everything dies. For most of us, *stillness* lives as an essence that is in the background of our lives, seldom noticed. But for Lilias, it's in the foreground, big-time.

This book is Lilias sharing her remarkable journey with us. It's not just her journey; it's ours, too. The ancient wisdom of yoga invites us, "Keep going. Stop not until the work is done." This book is Lilias's way of extending just such an invitation to us. She is someone who doesn't stop, who keeps going, and who is saying, "If I can do it, so can you."

Some people say that it takes courage to speak as Lilias is doing. I say it's the only thing that she can do. When we're true to ourselves, when we stop separating from what we know we need to do and say, we become the secret that Lilias is being; where we truly live from the heart of wisdom that comes with age. Just so, yoga is likened to being the two wings of a bird. One wing is love and the other is wisdom. Without either wing, this yoga bird can't fly and neither can we. It's delightful to witness Lilias in full flight with her two wings outstretched, saying to life, "Yes!" Listen now as she invites us to stretch our wings and say to life from the bottom of our hearts, "Yes!"

—Richard Miller, Ph.D.
Sebastopol, December 1, 2004

Acknowledgments

Heartfelt thanks to my husband, Bob, for his daily encouragement, support, love, and patient computer expertise. He is the wind beneath my wings.

Thanks to my sons and beautiful daughters-in-law, Michael, Jennifer, Matthew, and Leslie; and our precious grandchildren, Taylor, Ryan, Gabrielle, Sydney, Hunter, Maxwell, and Oliver.

Thank you and gratefulness to those great teachers who have inspired my journey. My root teacher, Sri Swami Chidananda, Sri Ramana Maharshi, Sri Goswami Kriyananda, Mr. T. K. V. Desikachar, Dr. Jean Klein, Dr. Jean Houston, Patricia Sun, Angela Farmer, Jean Bernard Rishi, Eckhart Tolle, and Ida Gryla.

Special thanks to Cincinnati Yoga Teachers Association and my students who have supported and cheered me on, especially Mary Fitzgerald, Julie Lusk, Angela Mc-Gowan, and Jeanne McGawain/Speier.

My deep thanks to Dr. Jean Houston and the Mystery School where I learned *The Body Poem*, a practice inspired by John Muir and given form by Elizabeth Cogburn. My explanation of "How Yoga Views the Stages of Life" in chapter 2 was inspired by this poem.

A deep bow and respect to Mr. B. K. S. Iyengar.

Leonard P. Goorian, producer, *Lilias, Yoga and You*, WCET-TV 48, Cincinnati, Ohio.

Circe Hamilton, photographer, who just happens to be my very dear niece, on her brilliant work!

Thank you to all my yoga buddies who remind me to laugh and walk with me on the journey, especially Richard Miller, Larry Payne, Mollie Lawson, Janie Maguire, Marti Glenn and Ken Bruer, Margaret and Burt Kramer, Stephan Cope, Nichala Joy Devi, and Jim Veltree and Jackie Jelinek in Toronto.

Our two brave, good-humored models for this book, Kevin Casey and Nancy Tatum (Glenmore Yoga Studio, Richmond, Virginia).

Everyone at Rodale Books, especially Jennifer Kushnier, editor, and Chris Gaugler, designer.

Rachelle Gardner, my editor, for her patience and ability to guide me through the labyrinth of this book.

Jeanne Fredericks, literary agent and friend.

Earth Angels Anne and Allen Zaring, who have made my journey on this planet easier, kinder, and full of generosity. India Supera and the Feathered Pipe Ranch in Helena, Montana. Sherry and Stewart Kahn. Debbie and Gary Goldman (NaturalJourneys.com).

Diane and Jay Dunkelman (Speaking of Women's Health).

Grace Hill, executive producer, *Lilias!*, CET-TV48.

Introduction: The Joy Is in the Journey

"From the yoga prospective, the raising of consciousness . . . is the ultimate definition of health."

—*International Journal of Yoga Therapy*

It was a sweltering January afternoon in Madras, India. My friends and I were in the monastery of Bhagavan Sri Ramakrishna, the great saint of modern India who lived in total God-consciousness.

Like the saints before him, he cared not for fame, power, or worldly prosperity. Ecstatic states were his norm. His mission was to prove that each individual soul is immortal and potentially divine. He saw all religions as many paths leading to the same goal: God is one. He taught that the way of self-knowledge (*Jnana*), combined with devotion (*Bhakti*), was a possibility for everyone who earnestly studied the teachings and who was willing to apply them in their daily lives.

In Madras it was easy to feel the sacredness at every turn, even in the Vedanta Book Shop where we were buying yoga books to lug back to the United States. I took a time-out and walked the cool halls of the monastery. Passing a small, cozy office, I saw a smiling, cheerful monk dressed in his orange robe, sitting behind his desk. He welcomed me in and invited me to sit down.

"What do you do?" he asked.

"I teach hatha yoga," I said.

At that moment, he became quiet and seemed to look at me from way in the back of his eyes. After some silence, the swami said in lilting English, "You know, we here in the East have taken yoga as far as we can go. Now it's up to you in the West to take it like a ball and run with it."

I was stunned. Here I was, sitting literally in the birthplace of yoga wisdom. How could we in the West possibly take the great message of Bhagavan Sri Ramakrishna, and other ancient luminaries, any further?

Today, as I recall that afternoon in Madras, I am touched by the swami's humility and kindness. How grateful I am that he shared this giant thought with me—a neophyte yoga teacher from Ohio. For as I look back over the last few decades of yoga in the Western world, I realize the swami was right. We have brought this ancient discipline up to the present, incorporating modern knowledge of the body's needs and limitations, while remaining true to the venerable roots of yoga.

Back in the '60s, the hatha yoga classes that I both took and taught were quite different than they are today. There might have been fifty students on an outdoor platform, and we were all doing the same yoga postures, the same way. Ages 20 to 80, all different sizes and shapes, many different fitness levels, yet we were not offered any variation in the way we did our postures. Few cautions were spoken. Everyone inhaled to the count of five and exhaled to the count of five. Each student tried to perform the postures perfectly—no matter if their bodies complained. There was not a sticky mat, Lili Pad, belt, blanket, or block in sight. (See Appendix A for explanations of these yoga tools.)

During those years, I began to notice something very troubling. I was developing injuries where before there were none. My friends could do magnificent scorpion arm balances, but in private told me how painful it was to sit straight in meditation. Almost everyone had a callus or puffy bruise on the back of the neck from doing shoulder stands on a bare floor. Perhaps you might have tried yoga and experienced similar discomfort. How could yoga postures, so highly touted as vehicles of physical and mental health, cause such discomfort?

In light of these disturbing questions, I knew there had to be a better way. Some problems, I could figure out for myself. I looked at the parts of the body as if they were links of a chain. If one link was weak, it affected the whole chain.

But I could only go so far with my own limited experience and observations. At just the right time, two brilliant yoga teachers came into my life, both of whom had studied for years with the great yogi Mr. B. K. S. Iyengar. Bernard Rishi and Angela Farmer gave me new insight about bodily alignment, the use of props, and ways to help students avoid injury. They also encouraged me to find my own voice as a teacher. I began to develop the teaching style that has come to be known as "Lilias yoga," a method that offers customized techniques and instructions for different body types and levels of fitness.

These days, many yoga teachers and reputable yoga schools are developing their own approaches to the practice based upon up-to-date information in anatomy, physiology, orthopedics, and other areas of medical science. Most good yoga teachers continually study to update their knowledge and increase their own skill. Much attention is paid to alignment, and students are instructed in safe approaches to every posture. The use of props is common to help students ease into postures, as well as to aid relaxation. As my swami from Madras predicted, over these last few decades, we have taken yoga to new levels.

This evolution has been not only in the physical realm; many Westerners are seeing how yoga also affects their spiritual, emotional, and mental selves. For me, yoga has been a journey into the many layers of Self, a profound tool for helping answer the question, "Who am I?"

I'm learning that part of getting to know yourself is being able to look at your life as both an inner and an outer journey. I picture my outer journey as horizontal—I'm walking along and I can see the horizon, and all the familiar landmarks along the way. It is what I'm doing and where I'm going. My inner journey is vertical—with no horizon, no specific goal. In this journey, I'm taking one step at a time. I don't look backward or forward, but experience each moment. I am not doing—I am being.

The joy in the journey does not necessarily come from reaching a goal or from attaining the summit. Joy comes from what transpires along the way. Probably the most fascinating thing I've discovered is that my yoga journey gets better with age. My friends chide me for using the "age" word in the title of this book. But the truth is, yoga *does* get better with age! And—age gets better with yoga. As I've gotten older, my physical, emotional, and spiritual needs have changed, and in many ways, yoga has helped me through those changes. My practice of yoga has changed, too, and now more than ever, I find that it is just what I need—in my body, my mind, and my soul.

Where are you on your journey? Have you reached an age—40, 50, 60—where you've decided you're going to get yourself in shape, once and for all? Or maybe you're just curious about yoga and wanted a book that didn't seem so targeted to thirty-somethings. Whatever your reason for picking up this book, I think you're going to find a gentle yet powerful approach to yoga that will naturally become an integral aspect of your life.

This is a sacred instant. Yesterday is done. Tomorrow is yet to come—there is only the present holy moment. Now is the time to take the first step toward the rest of your life. May I join you on your journey? Good. And now we begin.

Lillias!

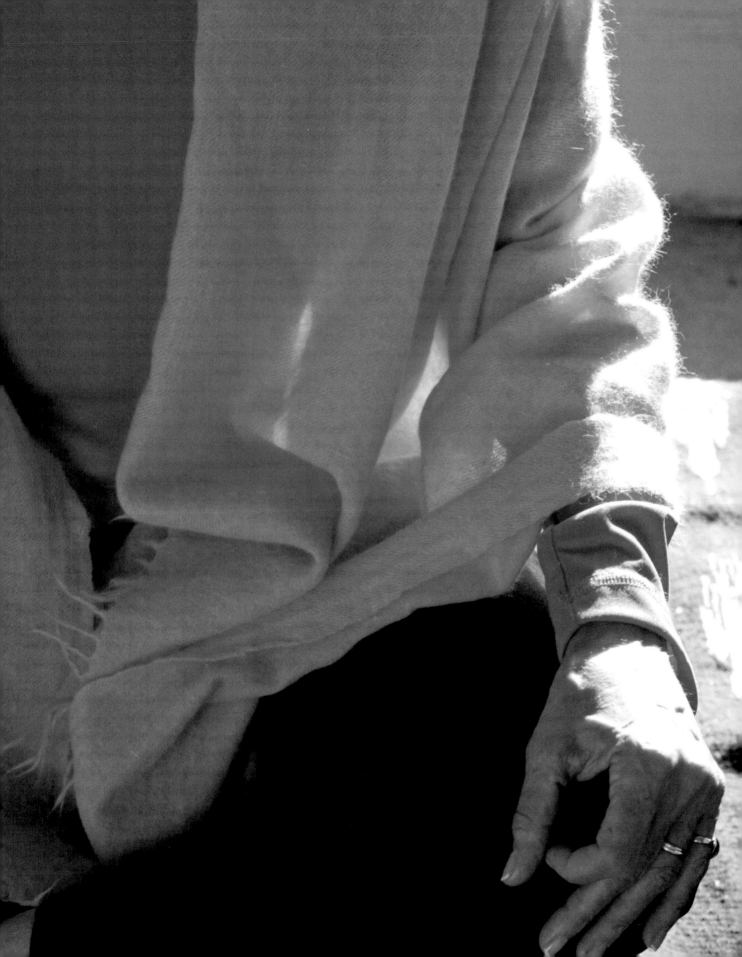

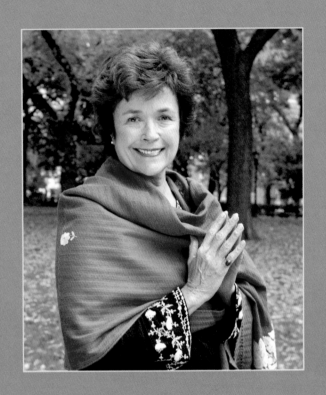

PART ONE

FROM THE HEART

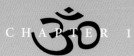

CHAPTER 1

WHAT IS LILIAS YOGA?

What is "Lilias yoga"? Folks ask me this question all the time, for good reason. Lilias yoga has appeared in *TV Guide* listings for years. The name originated with my television show, and as I developed my own particular style of teaching and became known for my gentle yet very effective approach, the name just stuck. Then, my first two books were *Lilias, Yoga and You* and *Lilias, Yoga and Your Life*—but honestly, there is no such thing as Lilias yoga.

In the ancient picture, no type of yoga was named after a human being (no Tom yoga, no Mary yoga, no Lilias yoga). But these days you hear all kinds of names before the word "yoga." The practice of yoga has been handed down and taught by such luminous yogis as Holy Master Swami Sivananda, B.K.S. Iyengar, and Mataji Indra Devi. I'm sure their enthusiastic and devoted students named particular yoga styles after their teachers—the teachers themselves didn't do it. These giants in the world of yoga all taught the same Down Dog pose. Any differences came from how the knowledge was interpreted, enhanced, and delivered.

I first began to establish the distinctive "Lilias" style of yoga in a darkened TV studio, teaching to a red light. But I never felt alone in that studio—I could always sense my unseen class. I pictured each student getting off the couch and sitting with me on the floor. Because I could not see my students, their comfort and safety in poses was always a prime concern. Going slowly through the postures, pulling them apart, and being clear about details and alignment became a style of teaching. The cameras used the body as a blackboard so the audience could see the poses and breathing from all angles. It was very important for me to explain everything I could about each pose and make sure I gave all the information needed to practice effectively and without injury. This was the beginning of Lilias yoga.

With all my talk about safety and comfort, though, I do have a confession to make. What ever possessed me to teach Headstand on television, I will *never* know. But I did. Talk about injury possibilities! Thank goodness, out of 500 taped yoga classes, I only once demonstrated this challenging posture. As chance would have it, that 5-minute Headstand became a very amusing moment in the classic movie *Being There.* Peter Sellers, in the character of Chauncey Gardiner, showed Shirley MacLaine how he had learned to stand on his head: while in bed, watching me on television. I think it's ironic that the one Lilias yoga moment that appeared in a major movie was an example of what Lilias yoga definitely is *not*: difficult and risky.

To understand where Lilias yoga fits into the big picture, I want to tell you a little about a core text of yoga philosophy called the *Yoga Sutra.* The *Yoga Sutra* explains that yoga is often compared to a big tree with eight limbs or branches, each limb representing a branch of yoga. Only one of these branches is *asana* (posture), the type of yoga that most of us in the United States are familiar with. It is actually a very small branch of this big tree. Yet, this small branch is a household word to many millions throughout the world. Some of the other branches are *pranayama* (breath control), *dhyana* (meditation), and *dharana* (concentration), which I'll also discuss in this book. Please don't be intimidated by all these unfamiliar words! Along the way, I'll be introducing you to Sanskrit terms, but I won't be expecting you to remember them.

All branches of yoga seek to achieve the same final goal: enlightenment. Hatha (pronounced haht-ha) uses the body, breath, and mind, your closest natural environment, as the perfect place to begin your study of the Self. The body, with all its layers, needs to be properly prepared to handle the increased energy of other stages of yoga, such as meditation. "Ha" in Sanskrit represents the sun energy; "tha," the lunar force. Hatha is the balancing and integration of those energies, helping them to move well throughout your body by means of the physical practice of yoga, through postures (asanas) and breathing (pranayama). Since the yoga I teach involves asana—incorporating the body, breath, and mind—it is a style of hatha yoga.

With so many "yogas" today, it's easy to get confused, and I want you to understand exactly what I'm teaching in this book—and what I'm not. Here, I'll describe just a few styles I am familiar with.

ANUSARA YOGA means "to step into the divine current of will." Developed by John Friend, this is a heart-opening hatha yoga practice. It is based on the three areas of attitude, alignment, and action.

ASHTANGA YOGA was developed by Sri K. Pattabhi Jois of Mysore, India. This is a continuous flowing practice, more physically intense than some styles, to build strength of mind and body.

POWER YOGA was developed by Beryl Bender Birch and is a Western adaptation of Ashtanga yoga. It is more athletic and often done with contemporary music.

VINIYOGA acknowledges the whole person, integrating postures, breath, and philosophy. Developed by T. K. V. Desikachar, this style is renowned for its therapeutic applications for assistance in recovery from injury and illness. Poses are customized to fit the needs of the practitioner.

SIVANANDA YOGA is based on the teachings of Holy Master Swami Sivananda of Rishikesh, India. Brought to the West in 1950, this system includes postures, breathing, chanting, and meditation, along with the study of yoga as it applies to one's life.

IYENGAR YOGA was developed by B. K. S. Iyengar of Pune, India, whose teachings are one of the most influential and well-known forms of hatha yoga. The focus is on precise alignment and subtleties within each asana. Using props helps the student adapt each pose to suit any body. To build strength, flexibility, and mind focus, the postures are held longer than they are in most traditions.

BIKRAM YOGA, known as "hot yoga," was founded by Bikram Choudhury and is practiced in a heated room. Twenty-six hatha yoga poses are done in a specific sequence, offering the opportunity to sweat and detox the body.

All of these approaches have much in common, yet they offer a wide variety of yoga study to fit all sorts of personalities. I have taken much of my teaching style from T. K. V. Desikachar, whose Viniyoga is known for being specific to the needs of the student, particularly anyone with special physical or emotional needs.

MISCONCEPTIONS

Lilias yoga has often been misunderstood, as has the entire discipline. *Lilias! Yoga and You* first aired on PBS in 1972. By the mid-1980s, the series was airing daily nationwide. I loved teaching yoga on TV, but I also really enjoyed getting out and teaching in person as often as possible.

My longtime friend and yoga buddy, psychologist Richard Miller, and I decided to hold a yoga workshop together near San Francisco. Today, yoga workshops are held every weekend all across the United States. But then, in the early 1980s, there were very few. Even though my show aired daily on KQED in San Francisco, I felt very insecure about people actually coming to the workshop. Wringing my hands, I voiced these concerns and worries to Richard as we drove to the studio: "Will anyone come? What if *nobody* comes?" Richard, in his quiet, humorous way, quickly guided my agitated thinking to a calmer, confident level.

Finally we pulled into the parking lot. We saw dozens of cars and what seemed like multitudes of people milling around the front door.

"Richard," I said joyously, "look at all the people who have come to take our workshop!"

As we got closer, we noticed something odd: everyone was carrying placards. They were not there to *take* the workshop; they were there to *picket* our workshop.

As we walked through the milling crowd, I peeked at the signs and leaflets being handed out. "YOGA—THE WORK OF THE DEVIL," in bold print. "YOGIS WORSHIP THE MONKEY GOD, HANUMAN, AND THE ELEPHANT GOD, GANESHA." It felt shocking and hurtful to come face-to-face with so many misunderstandings and outright lies about yoga.

That day, many yoga students did push

through the picketers and attend our workshop. But the experience left me with more questions than answers. I knew in my bones that yoga is not the work of the devil. (I also loved the round, friendly elephant called Ganesha, whose job was to remove obstacles in life, and I felt inspired by Hanuman, so devoted to the service of God.) But I still wasn't absolutely, positively clear about what yoga is and is not. How did yoga fit in with my Christian roots? Slowly, answers would come, as yoga concepts and truths became integral to my own personal experience, not just something I had read in a book. I will share many of these answers with you in the following chapters and show

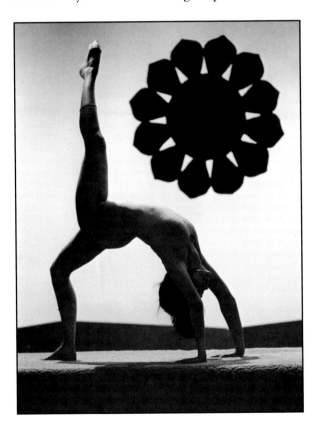

This is me practicing Upward-Facing Bow on the PBS set of *Lilias! Yoga and You,* 1972.

you how to come to your own conclusions as well.

Yoga has long been associated with the Hindu religious traditions. It is true that yoga emerged from India as a set of practices with spiritual content; however, it is not married to any particular religious tradition.

Yoga means to join—the unification of two things. For some, this means joining hands to toes in a forward bend. Others understand it to mean joining the human heart with the heart of God. Either way is correct. It is a process. Whether you're touching hands to feet or reaching for God, there must be movement. This movement is yoga.

The physical, mental, and spiritual benefits of yoga are well documented. Hatha yoga is practiced in Buddhist and Christian monasteries and convents around the world. It is also a vital part of Dr. Dean Ornish's hospital program for reversing heart disease.

Yoga is not about adopting any particular set of beliefs but about coming to *know* through your own experience. It is not about blindly following anything or anyone, but it is about assisting *you* on your chosen path. Nothing in yoga competes with any religious pathway or system of belief. Yoga is the science and study of the Self. It is a vehicle for inner growth and development. Yoga emphasizes the doing and the practice. It can be adapted to fit every body, no matter what size, shape, age, or physical condition—all are welcome!

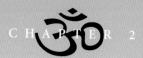

CHAPTER 2

HOW YOGA VIEWS THE STAGES OF LIFE

The one-size-fits-all approach to yoga practice has never felt comfortable to me. The idea of adapting yoga to the individual, however, rather than adapting the individual to the practice, feels practical and natural. Adapting postures is not new. It is actually part of the ancient tradition of yoga, especially Viniyoga (see below). Developing and adapting a personal yoga practice means respectfully taking into consideration age, health issues, gender, capacities, and activities.

The Viniyoga approach divides one's life into stages, like following the movements of the sun as it travels across the sky. Sunrise represents childhood; midday represents midlife; and sunset, old age.

We can also divide life into seasons, recognizing that as humans we are not only aging, we are *evolving* and growing until the day we take our last breath. In springtime, new life comes into being. The sultry heat of summer is a time of growth. Autumn, with its richness and ripening, feels light after the heaviness of summer. Winter is a time of maturity, of knowing, and closure. And then, finally, once again it is spring.

Each season has its own corresponding element, animal power, and gift teaching. While these may not resonate with some, I find they're creative, poetic ways of connecting with the various aspects of the Self at this juncture of the journey. The animal power is a metaphor to help you see the most powerful and positive characteristics of this life stage, and the gift teachings represent the nuggets of wisdom we struggle to learn during this season. Whatever your age, as you read through the phases in the following pages, let each season, part of the day, element, animal power, and gift teaching flow through you.

THE FIRST PHASE

DIRECTION: East

SEASON: Spring, a time of budding, rebirth

DAY PART: Dawn

ELEMENT: Air

ANIMAL POWER: The eagle, the long view of your life

GIFT TEACHING: The power and daring to take the first step

This stage covers about the first 25 years of life. Someone in this phase enjoys a hatha yoga practice designed to promote the development of body and mind. Even young children can participate in half-hour classes that consist mostly of relaxation full of imagery. Postures can be renamed to make them friendly and easy to relate to: Cobra Pose becomes Sneaky Snake; Standing Forward Bend might be Inchworm. A fun way to approach relaxation would be to call it Melting Ice-Cream Cone.

Throughout the teens and into our 20s, we're still in the sunrise part of life. Our practice is balanced; we find some of the "hot" or more athletic practices fun and challenging (such as Bikram or Power Yoga). People in this phase usually need to strengthen and lengthen shoulder and lower-back muscles, in hopes of avoiding the back and wrist pain that often come with a budding career and long hours of sitting at a desk. Fully experiencing proper breathing is a vital, inexpensive, portable tool for managing stress. Learning how to consciously relax can open the door to making meditation part of your life.

THE SECOND PHASE

DIRECTION: South

SEASON: Summer

DAY PART: High noon

ELEMENT: Fire

ANIMAL POWER: Mountain lion, graceful and elegant; mouse, innocence, the detailed view of your life.

GIFT TEACHING: Thy will be done

The high noon of life covers roughly the years between 25 and the 40s. This is a great time to experience all types of hatha yoga classes. In this stage, we find what's best for us and our lifestyle. It is a challenging time of trying to squeeze a yoga practice into a busy life of carrying out household responsibilities, raising a family, paying bills, sometimes caring for aging parents. A well-structured practice can promote stability on every level. Today there are specialized classes for pregnant women, stressed-out business people, and athletes, as well as many excellent videos to strengthen the home practice.

THE THIRD PHASE

DIRECTION: West

SEASON: Autumn, colorful, beautiful change

DAY PART: Afternoon

ELEMENT: Water

ANIMAL POWER: The snake, a time of shedding, letting go

GIFT TEACHING: Yes! to life (L'Chaim in the Hebrew tradition)

I had a challenging time coming up with a day-part name for us midlife yogis. The truth is, we are somewhere between high noon and sunset. So I've named our day part afternoon, which covers the ages from 50 to 70-something. It is the main focus of this book.

Many midlifers are restarting their yoga practice. Today, those 50 and beyond are not what people of the same age were 100 years ago. We look, act, and feel younger, and hopefully we're healthier than our ancestors. For some, it's a time of new beginnings, of redefining what's real and important in life. It can be a season of shedding, downsizing, and letting go of stuff—trinkets, emotional baggage, an outdated self-concept, or children heading off to college.

Many find this to be an unexpected era of discovery and begin to delve into the ancient question, who am I? We might feel like going inward, practicing relaxation skills on and off the mat. It's a time to heed the inner call to get on with spiritual homework, setting aside time for meditation and spiritual reading. For women, a hatha practice to strengthen bone health and balance emotions can ease the travel through menopause. Midday men and women are often surprised and awed by their ability to

progress and achieve challenging postures formerly perceived as impossible. A new sense of confidence develops.

THE FOURTH PHASE

DIRECTION: North

SEASON: Winter

DAY PART: Sunset into night

ELEMENT: Earth, snow-capped mountains of maturity

ANIMAL POWER: Buffalo, abundance, self-giving, plenty for all

GIFT TEACHING: Stillness; the giving away; non-attachment to the results of our creative actions

The sunset phase covers the senior years, roughly 70 and beyond. All our preparation for this moment pays off now. Our goal is to stay active, mentally and physically. Even though the afternoon stage of life is swiftly closing, it's never too late to begin yoga! Progress can be dramatic: walking, gardening, and even sleep come easier.

This is a time to keep yoga practice simple and include weight-bearing postures to keep our back, hips, and legs strong. Practice getting down onto the floor from a chair, and up off the floor with the help of a chair. Practice standing tall against the wall and balancing on one foot, keeping a chair close by for help in balance. Simple balancing poses strengthen the "wobble" muscles, helping us keep our balance getting in and out of the shower or during a golf swing.

Practicing relaxation reconnects us to our natural contentment and wisdom. *Pranayama*, our breathing practice, becomes a powerful tool for maintaining a healthy, energetic body and clearing and quieting the mind. For those who have a feeling for it, taking time to deepen our spiritual connection through prayer and meditation becomes all-important.

UNDERSTANDING MY LIFE in the framework of these seasons allows me to see the value in each phase. As we get older, it can be easy to give in to hopelessness as we finally recognize our mortality. But when we understand that our afternoon and sunset years have a value and a purpose all their own, we gain a new appreciation for these years. Suddenly we desire to live them for all they're worth!

I've found that to make the most of the second half of my life, I've had to stop being afraid of looking inward. When we become willing to stop, be reflective, and look within, we find that each of us has many layers to ourselves that we've never had time to explore. The later years offer a perfect opportunity to change our focus from the external, material, and physical world to that which is unseen and harder to perceive.

The yoga journey on which I am taking you is meant to help you gain access to parts of yourself you may never have thought about. I'm going to approach yoga in a way that you won't find in other books. I'm going to try to help you gain a new perspective on aging, while teaching you yoga postures and methods of stretching and relaxing that are perfectly suited for your stage of life.

So before we dive into our practice of yoga, we need to prepare for this journey. The next section will begin to explain what I mean when I talk about the Self having "layers," and we'll also look at a few provisions we'll need to take with us on this yoga voyage.

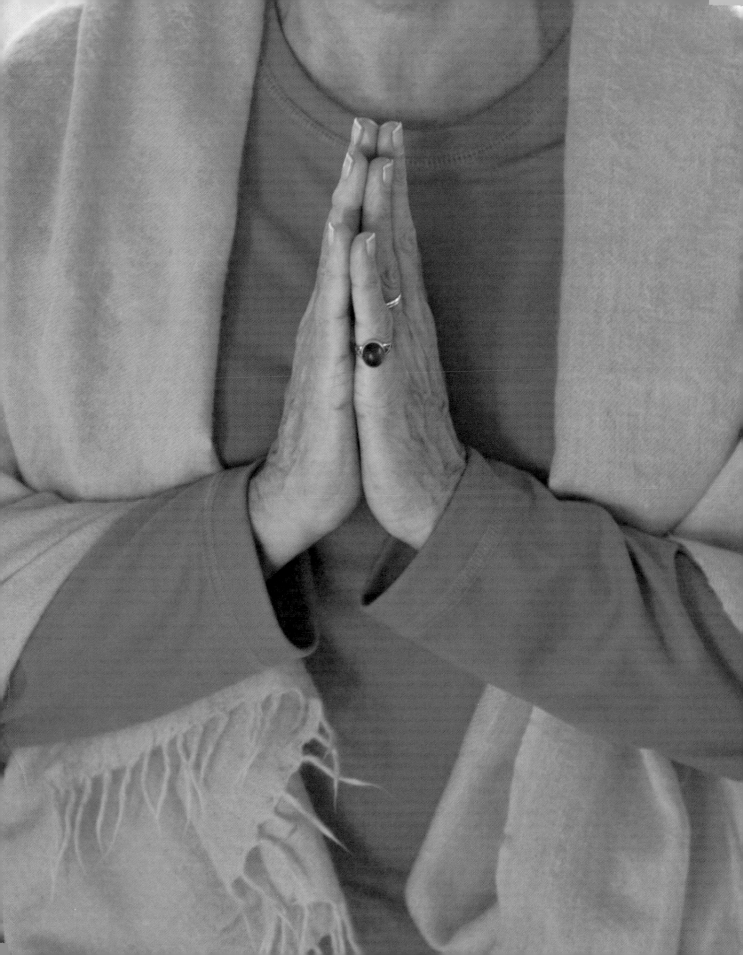

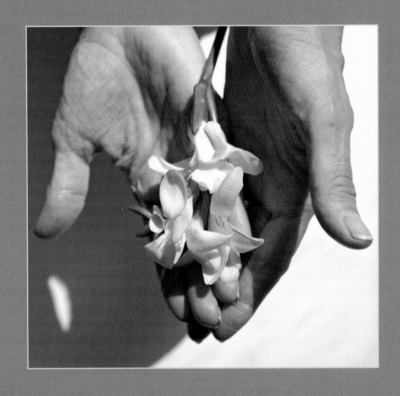

PART TWO

PREPARING FOR
THE JOURNEY

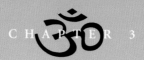

CHAPTER 3

YOUR MULTILAYERED SELF

I s this it? Is this all there is?" I had lots of *things*, including a boat on Long Island Sound and two golden retrievers. Why wasn't I happy?

Perhaps it was the realization that I wasn't getting any younger. So I began my version of spiritually "working" on myself: marital therapy, parenting therapy, sex therapy, mother-daughter therapy, workshops to heal the inner child, yoga intensives for the perfect outer body.

In the midst of all this scurrying around, finding time for myself alone in the form of an afternoon nap seemed like an indulgence. Little did I know that one nap in particular would change my life.

Half awake and half dreaming, I sat bolt upright in bed. As I looked around, something strange was going on. I was sitting in a bed covered with steaming brown mounds of fecal matter: stalactites of brown feces hung from my bedroom ceiling, dripping huge brown piles on my bed. I sat still, not daring to move an inch. Suddenly a voice boomed loud enough to fill the room and my whole body, "Clean up your act!" Instantly I knew exactly to what the voice was referring: my so-called work on myself.

"But I am working so-o-o hard on myself," I answered, whining defensively (and thinking of all those therapies and workshops). "I really am."

The voice turned up the decibels and boomed louder, *"Clean up your act!"* I felt like I had put my finger in an electrical socket. Pouting in silence, I sat, feeling embarrassed and vulnerable that something from another dimension had seen through the veneer of my "act," and cared enough to blast through my defenses in hopes that I would hear.

I drifted back to sleep, allowing time for the revolting vision to dissolve. The echo of the booming message delivered with so much tough love would continue to vibrate and deepen for years to come. It was not that my time and efforts to "work on myself" were superficial or worthless. Quite the contrary. Different therapies, especially those intense years spent in traditional psychotherapy, were pivotal in healing past deep emotional wounds. But that dramatic vision was calling me to truly "get my s--t together" before it was too late!

"Clean up your act" began to mean different things. It was time to move into the deeper housekeeping mode we used to call spring cleaning. I needed to bring out the blankets and rugs of my Self, hang them in the sun, use my spiritual muscles to give them a big shake, and watch the dust fly.

It was time to let go of the dust bunnies of *restlessness* and *discontent*; time to declutter and give up useless strategies for feeling safe and in control. I needed to uncover my capacity to stay *present* in all of life's conditions and shine up my courage to love without strings, guarantees, or requirements. The time had come to stop trying to change myself; after all, when spring cleaning we don't move to a new house. Instead I needed to clear away all the dirt and begin acknowledging myself for who I really am. *Self-acceptance* would be the healing force for positive change.

Part of "cleaning up the act" was to stop acting as if the pure light of the High Self did not exist. But how would I dig through the layers and discover the truest part of me? In my reading, I encountered an ancient Eastern concept that would lead me on a lifelong journey of self-discovery that continues to this day.

THE KOSHAS

Have you exercised your physical body lately? Chances are, yes, you've been to the gym, taken a walk, or done your yoga practice. But have you exercised your subtle body or your causal body? I can just hear you asking, "What in the world are you talking about?"

In traditional yoga texts, the layers of our selves are called *maya koshas*. Literally, *maya* means "illusion" and a *kosha* is a body or sheath (a covering). So the ancients conceptualized the Self as not one body but five distinct "bodies" layered on top of one another that cover the pure light of the highest Self. Each body is a distinct maya kosha, or kosha for short.

Each kosha is made up of increasingly finer energy vibrations as you move inward. We can *see* the physical body, but the other four bodies are energy states invisible to the naked eye. If you pay attention, you can easily sense and feel their presence within you.

The five bodies form a covering for the pure Self, or light within. These sheaths are often compared to layers of an onion that, over time, become so thick and hardened that they completely cover what's within. They become obstacles that hinder our way to experiencing the sacred light.

The inner light is the one constant; it does not change. Wind cannot blow it out. Water cannot drown it nor fire burn it. Everything else changes—our aging bodies, nature surrounding us—all is in constant change, but our inner light stays the same.

Some of us have trouble conceptualizing this inner light. It's not a strictly religious concept, although every religion has a name for it. Some people think of this deepest part of us as the soul. Others call it the God within, or their highest Self.

However we refer to it, at some point in our lives we discover we cannot neglect it. But how do we find it in the first place? In order to gain access to our inner light, we must exercise, clean up, breathe life into, strengthen, tone, and relax each of our bodies—our koshas.

At birth, kosha layers are translucent and thin—soft, pliable membranes. The inner light easily shines through newborn babies and young children. I have known many children, including me when I was young, who experienced easy access to the loving presence of light from within. I called it my friend. When things were lonely, difficult, and chaotic during my childhood, especially at night, I could connect with a soothing, calm, loving presence in the center of my chest. Sometimes a voice would gently offer guidance and wisdom. Like almost everyone, I lost touch with this part of myself as I grew older. But understanding the koshas has been instrumental in bringing me full circle, back to a place where I am familiar with my purest Self.

In parts three through seven of this book, I'm going to take you on a yoga journey through your koshas. Right now, I just want to give you a brief overview. The concept of koshas provides you with the map, a starting point, to explore this unfamiliar inner territory of your Self.

So let's begin with your physical body, known as *anna-maya-kosha*. At least we can *see* it! We use the yoga postures—the asanas—as a way to reconnect with and listen to the physical body. Often we take for granted the health of this body until it talks back and insists we pay attention.

Your second body is your energy/breathing body, *prana-maya-kosha*. This breath body is also easy to forget or take for granted. But imagine someone tying a 50-pound weight to your feet and pushing you into a swimming pool. As you sink to the bottom, what will be your next thought? A new car? How the stock market's doing? No-o-o, I think your next thought will be *I have to breathe!* Becoming aware of your flow of breathing is the first step in contacting your breathing body and an avenue into awareness of the deeper koshas.

Your third body is that of the mind, senses, and emotions, *mano-maya-kosha*. Thoughts, feelings, and all that you perceive from your five senses reside within this kosha. In our modern-day stressful society, this body tends to be knotted with stress, restlessness, and overload. Practicing the postures and breathing techniques of yoga is one of the best ways to keep this body in balance. Later in the book, I'll share easy, practical, balanced ways to stretch and exercise, loosening the knots of stress and soothing the restless mind.

Your fourth body—subtler still—is called *vijnana-maya-kosha* and means "wisdom body." When this kosha is underdeveloped, you have a hard time making decisions, possess seemingly very little willpower, and are continually the victim of your own poor judgment. Recognizing the value of expanding your self-awareness is a first step to contacting your wisdom body. Accessing the high mind and wisdom can be enormously fun, deeply strengthening, and creative.

Your fifth body is *ananda-maya-kosha*. *Ananda* means "bliss." Here is the subtlest body, the thinnest veil, which stands between ordinary awareness and the state of stillness, peace, bliss, and the light existing within us all. For the vast majority of humans, this sheath is totally underdeveloped. In the past, it seemed like experiencing the bliss body was reserved for saints and sages, but this is definitely changing. The practice of relaxation, breathing, and keeping a heart-centered practice will help awaken the bliss body.

Each of these bodies, or koshas, is a very real presence within you, and I'm sure you'll find it exciting to get in contact with them. Throughout the rest of this book, I'll guide you on this inward journey through the layers of yourself. You'll learn yoga postures, breathing methods, relaxation exercises, and meditation techniques that will help you on this inward excursion. But we need to do one more thing before embarking: We must for a moment switch our focus to what we'll need to take with us. In the next chapter, I'll help you "pack a bag" with just the right provisions for this yoga expedition.

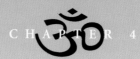

CHAPTER 4

WHAT DO YOU NEED FOR THE JOURNEY?

You've realized by now that we're doing more than learning a few yoga postures. While you may have become interested in yoga because you felt the need to keep your bones strong and muscles in shape, I've learned from experience that we miss a lot when we pay attention only to our physical selves. In order to practice the postures of yoga to their fullest effect, we need to be aware of our *whole* selves—inside and out. So we're taking a journey inward.

As for all journeys, we need to pack a bag. This journey is a little different, however—I won't need warm socks or an extra turtleneck. So what will I absolutely, positively need to help navigate the misty inner layers of Self? Here is the short list of provisions I think we all need to carry:

- Witness self
- One-pointed attention
- Detachment
- Nonviolence
- Contentment
- Self-study
- Relaxation
- Meditation

Each one of the above could be considered a spiritual muscle. As with all muscles, you need to use 'em or lose 'em. Each time you ponder, con-template, or reflect, you are strengthening your spiritual muscles. When you begin to practice the postures of yoga, these tools will assist you. But best of all, you can choose to carry them out of the yoga room and into your daily life.

THE WITNESS SELF
(Sakshin)

The mystics of the past encourage us to "close the outer eyes, so that the inner eye can open."

Today, let me introduce you to the friend that walks with you on your journey. Some call it your witness self. To others, it's known as the observer or witness consciousness. The yogis gave the witness a lovely Sanskrit name—

sakshin. I call it one of my best friends, and it is a pleasure for me to share this friendship with you.

The witness is centered in the present moment, with no memories of the past or concerns for the future. It is untouched by the approval or disapproval of others. It is self-accepting in both failure as well as success.

You might imagine that befriending your witness is impossible and maybe sounds schizophrenic, but it's not. (I promise.) In fact, you've probably met your witness many times before, but just weren't aware of it.

We'll travel with our witness through all the following chapters, but for this moment in time, try the exercise below to get you started.

It is not difficult to contact your witness. The challenge is staying connected. It's like holding hands with my wiggly four-year-old granddaughter as we go through the Kroger parking lot. She just wants to run off and play. I have to work hard at keeping those little fingers connected to mine.

With regular practice, your witness will strengthen and become a quiet, almost effortless presence in your life. Richard Rosen, in his book *The Yoga of Breath*, says, "When the witness

AN EXERCISE TO CONNECT WITH YOUR WITNESS

BEGIN WITH YOUR CLOSEST NATURAL ENVIRONMENT—your body. While sitting in a chair, close your eyes. In your mind, step back from your body, and view it like a big puzzle or painting in which you want to scan your awareness over the whole surface all at once.

Then read the following sentences slowly, pausing after each one. Sit back in your chair . . . feel the warmth of your skin as it touches the back of the chair . . . bring your awareness to the inside of your head . . . go way into the back (cave) of your skull, eyes closed, gaze outward . . . you are looking into the back of your face as if it were a Halloween mask. Feel your brow smooth as silk . . . feel where your eyelids touch . . . upper lid . . . lower lid . . . become aware of your nostrils . . . how the air flows in . . . and out . . . . warm . . . cool . . . now feel where your two lips touch . . . feel the length of your lips. Ask yourself, "Who is watching?" The answer: the witness.

Do this exercise several times a day if you can, and in between, try to keep that witness with you.

shines a light on the unnecessary and unhealthy doing-somethings of the surface self and surface breather, they immediately lose some of their potency, and grip, and so suffering is weakened."

There are some qualities about your new friend that you might like to know. Number one is major!

1. Your witness *judges not* (lest ye be judged). The nonjudgmental witness practices self-observation without criticism. As you enter the door of yoga class—even if it's your living room—make it a habit to hang your judge's black robe on an imaginary hook. (As you leave, choose if you wish to put it back on.) This means there is no value judgment on "how well" you perform yoga postures and no pressure to compete.

2. There is absolutely nothing your witness cannot see. No shame. No shadow. No embarrassment. No fear.

3. Experiencing your witness is not an exercise in thinking. To the contrary, we actually allow the whole body to feel the vibrations, the shimmering of sensations, as they filter through the different koshas. Witness is an essence of who we are.

4. Witness neither slumbers nor sleeps but remains awake, present, and potentially available within every human being. Its sacred ground need only be recognized, cultivated, protected, and celebrated.

Stephen Cope, psychologist, author, and master yogi, says in his book *Yoga and the Quest for the True Self*, "Contemporary Western psychologists, like yogis, believe that if this 'seer' is insufficiently developed, we will suffer and become overidentified with thoughts and feelings. Without the still point of the witness we feel fragmented and fragile." I like introducing you to your witness self early on in this book because from this moment on, sakshin will accompany you on every aspect of your journey through the five koshas, your yoga practice, and hopefully, your life.

ONE-POINTED ATTENTION
(Dharana)

Packing lightly is not my strong suit (please pardon the pun!), but I know my packing list will include one-pointed attention, or concentration. Single-pointed concentration has been given a Sanskrit name, *dharana*. Try it out the next time you brush your teeth. See how long you can stay present and focused on the two-minute act of teeth brushing. Notice how many times your mind wants to jump from one topic to another.

We live in a culture that trains us well in multitasking. Performing more than one task at a time might seem like an efficient use of energy, but it really is not. It might appear that I can drive and talk on my cell phone, but to accomplish this, my poor brain must run back and forth, and I end up not doing either very well.

Scientific studies show that multitasking asks the brain to function beyond its capacity. Our good friend the brain cannot process more than one piece of information at a time. It actually goes on overload with so many multitasking demands. When this happens, it sends an SOS—*Help!*—to the adrenals, which then release adrenaline. Many of us live in a continual state of overload. Prolonged release of adrenaline can lead to numerous problems, including trouble sleeping, clinical depression, and anxiety.

Don't underestimate or devalue the power of your own dharana. As you develop your one-pointed attention, you'll find yourself less distracted, agitated, or scattered. Your ability to focus on a given task will grow stronger, and you'll find yourself being not only more effective but also more peaceful.

Meditation, even in its early stages, will give you the experience of dharana. Meditation can help you quiet the restless, wandering mind that has been traveling at breakneck speeds, weaving from lane to lane, observing no traffic regulations whatsoever. Even if you don't meditate, you have numerous opportunities to practice your concentration. As you stand at the sink washing dishes, try to pay attention only to what you're doing, without letting your mind wander. Notice the unique shape of each dish and utensil; feel the sensation of the water on your hands; listen for the subtle crackle of the soap bubbles.

While it may seem difficult (and it is for all of us!), this type of practice is valuable in strengthening your concentration in all areas of your life.

Teaching yoga in a darkened studio quickly brought to my awareness the weakness of my concentration. TV studios are quiet while filming, yet there is always movement or low talking behind the cameras. Each day I would give a class to the impersonal red light of the TV camera, hoping that my words would flow naturally and with ease. But every time there was a sound or movement, my mind would wander dangerously off course. Panicked, I'd begin to reach deep inside and hold on to concentration for dear life. The action of reaching inward, digging deep, and holding on to the train of thought again and again began to strengthen the dharana "muscle." This mind of mine still wanders, but I feel more prepared. Today they could hold a line dance behind the cameras, and, hopefully, I would still sit there, in one-pointed concentration, talking directly to the red light and my viewers.

DETACHMENT
(Aparigraha)

It was time to downsize, to sell our home of 32 years. Home: where we raised our two boys, now married with children of their own. Home of 32 Christmases and Thanksgivings. Home with *big* closets filled with clothes that *maybe* I'll be thin enough to wear; bureau drawers with enough yoga T-shirts and tights for an army of yogis. Kitchen drawers stuffed with utensils. Library shelves heavy with my 40-year collection of beloved yoga books.

I'm not great at dealing with change. Change makes me feel unsettled and anxious. The new home was smaller, with very small closets and virtually no bookshelves. The whole project felt painful and overwhelming.

Deep down I knew it was time to sit with the uncomfortable feelings that arose with wanting to attach, hold, grasp onto things. I probably needed to explore my discomfort with change, too.

Then it dawned on me. This move was giving me the opportunity to practice the yoga of non-attachment—*aparigraha*. My first lesson was that detachment does not mean disinterest. I was being given a chance to simplify and streamline my life on many levels. This would take energy, interest, and letting go of attachment to the end results.

My mantra quickly became "If you haven't worn it in three years, let it go!" Finding agencies through whom I could give my stuff to the less fortunate became a pleasure. Family china that I covet could be mentally given away to my wonderful daughters-in-law. All my beloved yoga books now have a new home in the Ram Dass Library at the Omega Institute in Rhinebeck, New York.

Years later, I still have a few unpacked boxes, as well as twinges of soft regret about what I've

let go. But with the iron chain of grasping finally severed, I have been able to put down the heavy burden. And with that comes the peace of detachment. This inner peace—peace of mind, soul, and spirit—is the reason we practice non-attachment.

Rarely is detachment achieved once and for all. For me it is moment-to-moment and day-to-day. I'm still learning to keep a watchful inner eye of interest without grasping on to desires and outcomes.

One of the strangest lessons in attachment came to me in the form of hair. Yes, my hair! In the early '70s, my *Lilias! Yoga and You* PBS television years, I grew my hair into a very long braid. It became sort of a trademark, the long braid and pink leotard. But as we moved into the 1980s, there came a stirring in me to cut it. Some part of me wanted to let go, get serious, move on, and grow up. To this day I encounter yoga folks who ask me, "Why did you cut your hair? What did you do with the braid? Save it?"

No, I didn't save it. But I did learn that, male or female, you are not your hair! The real you is within and is far more beautiful than anyone can imagine.

After attachments to hair, clothing, and cars (remember the gentleman who was buried in his Cadillac?) come the really knotty issues. These are the attachments to family, children, animals, youth, or the idea that "I am this body." Attachments can be so visceral that to let go feels like letting go of life itself.

If you want to experiment with detachment, try starting with the small, easy stuff, like clothes and unimportant objects. Challenge yourself: Sometime this week, go through your house and find 20 objects to either throw, put, or give away. Then go through your closets and drawers. Find 10 items of clothing to relinquish. Once the stuff is gone, pay attention to how you are feeling. Are you stuck in sadness and regret? Your "detach muscle" definitely needs strengthening. Congratulations for taking on this difficult exercise! If you are feeling a little lighter, despite twinges of regret, you're starting to experience the benefits of detachment.

As you get better at this, you'll want to work into stickier, more complex attachments. Keep your witness at your side and humor in your heart! Detachment takes practice and time. It's easier with a soft, lighthearted attitude.

Sometimes I can ease into letting go of painful emotional attachments by offering them up to a higher power. Perhaps I'm angry with someone but consider it righteous anger: I'm right and they're wrong. I'm usually tempted to hold on to my anger—after all, I'm the one who's right. I know I need to detach from my anger, but I can't figure out how. I don't know where to put it. So I offer it up to God, Higher Power, Great Spirit. This sacred time-honored method helps loosen my cementlike hold. It allows me to release the fruits of my actions, desires, fears, and doubts.

Let me say again that detachment is not cal-

AN EXERCISE TO STRENGTHEN YOUR DETACH MUSCLE

SIT QUIETLY, EYES CLOSED. WATCH YOUR BREATHING FOR A FEW MOMENTS. Connect with your quiet, still, inner presence. Now silently offer the picture and the feelings of wanting, intending, doing, or whatever you're trying to get free of, to that energy that feels most essential to your life. Once you make your offering to a higher power, remind yourself that you truly have let it go. The temptation is to reach up and snatch it back. So, again, make your offering . . . watch it dissolve . . . then linger in that nurturing, peaceful space you've created within your Self.

You might picture the thing you're letting go of as a kite. Slowly let out the string, and watch the kite float higher and higher. At some point, you have to let go of the string.

lous indifference or impersonal disinterest. It is a day-to-day practice, using skillful thinking and actions. The next time you feel attachment's grip, make an offering and keep working with the small stuff. Imagine all fears and attachment dissolving, creating more space for stillness and love within. When we're faced with grief, loss, or failure, our practice in detachment becomes a lifeline that can move us out of acute suffering into something close to peacefulness and ease.

NONVIOLENCE
(Ahimsa)

The habit and practice of being kind, first to yourself, then to others, is known as *ahimsa*. It's sometimes referred to as nonviolence or noninjury. Ahimsa suggests a deep commitment to not causing pain to anyone or anything through thoughts, words, or actions. The wise sages of yoga teach us that everything we think, say, or do needs to be in harmony with nonviolence.

Mahatma Gandhi asserted, "Ahimsa is an attribute of the soul to be practiced by everyone in all affairs of life." Ahimsa is the golden rule: "Do unto others as you wish done unto you."

Critical, judgmental thoughts of yourself (and others), even striving for perfection in yoga poses, is a subtle form of violence and does harm. Consciously finding little things to love, about yourself and others, warms and heals the heart and creates contentment.

Ahimsa is thinking charitable thoughts about

yourself (and your neighbor). It is a practice that begins with you. Remember? Charity begins at home. The next time you catch yourself thinking "I'm so fat" or "She's so mean," remember ahimsa. Consciously change your thought: "I'm lovable the way I am, and I'm working toward a goal" or "She must be having a bad day; I wonder how I can help."

Later in the book, as we begin to practice yoga postures, I will remind you to approach each pose with ahimsa. This will help you form the nonharming habit. It's a great practice, easily translated into your everyday life.

CONTENTMENT
(Santosha)

Friends told me to my face how difficult I was to sit next to in *satsang* (group meditation). Each time I tried to sit quietly on the meditation cushion, restlessness and irritability rolled out of my body in great waves. Even my yoga classmates felt my discontent.

What does it mean to be contented? It's a feeling of being satisfied right where you are, with exactly what you have. In our society, discontent usually stems from wanting more; it's like an itch that can never be scratched. We want to be richer or thinner or more popular or more successful; we want to have more things, experience a more exciting life. We want our spouse to be more attentive and our children to be more obedient. Whoever we are and whatever we have, it's not enough. Personally, I am always wanting to be a better person, practice yoga better, be a better wife, mother, and grandmother. There's nothing wrong with wanting to improve! But never being satisfied is the hallmark of discontent.

Feeling peaceful and at ease is a huge challenge for all of us living on this media-filled planet. Our entire culture is based on the desire for more—and we are bombarded with messages from morning till night that tell us we're somehow not good enough. In fact, I would have to say that our whole economy—capitalism itself—is based on our collective discontent.

If that weren't enough, our media also saturate us with every bad, ugly, selfish, cruel act throughout the world. We can be overwhelmed by it and begin to think, what's the point? We'd feel guilty if we actually experienced contentment in such an awful world.

Now, I admit I'm not going to solve the whole contentment problem in this little yoga book. I just want to call your awareness to your own level of contentment or discontent. If you're going to journey within yourself, it's one of the things you'll need to face. In addition, practicing yoga postures while consumed with discontent is missing the point.

Spend a moment contemplating contentment. What are you satisfied with? In what areas of your life are you chronically unhappy? The antidote to discontent is gratitude. What are you grateful for? When you embrace thankfulness for the things, people, and circumstances of your life, contentment grows. Contentment contains the fullness of life and a droplet of bliss. Everything of beauty, of meaning, is held within contentment.

If you feel a little unplugged from your contentment connection, the practice of meditation and relaxation skills given in the next few chapters will help you clear negative debris that separates us all from *santosha* (contentment). In time you will experience a softening and mellowing of your personality. Rough edges will automatically smooth out. You will feel it, and your family will benefit from it. It's easy to see why mystics of past and present considered contentment vital to pack for life's journey.

SELF-STUDY
(Svadhyaya)

One of my early milestones came years ago, as I approached the backstage entrance to a Philadelphia television studio. It was shrouded in the dense late-afternoon winter shadows. A lonely light hung above the door. I was a bundle of nerves, about to go live on national television to playfully teach yoga to megastars Anthony Quinn, Mike Douglas, and baseball's affable Joe Garagiola.

Feeling awkward and out of place, I reached the dimly lit stage door. Out of the shadows came an old woman in tattered clothing, lumbering quickly toward me. Disappointed not to see a famous face, she squinted at me, then thrust an

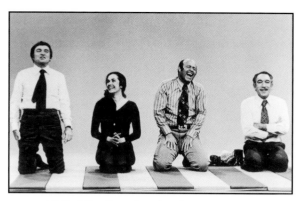

1972: Mike Douglas, Joe Garagiola, and
Anthony Quinn had fun trying yoga!

autograph book into my chest. With a cackle, she said, "Hey lady, are you *some*body?" In slow motion, I heard my thoughts: "No, I'm not a *some*body, but I'm not *no*body either." Ever since then, I've tried to answer the question, if I'm not a *some*body, and I'm not a *no*body . . . who am I?"

That question has been the catalyst for me to spend years cultivating the art of self-study, or *svadhyaya*. It is the art of introspection, of exploring who we are. One of the ways we do this is by being aware of our thoughts and objectively observing our actions. (There's our witness Self again!)

For centuries, spiritual greats from all traditions have led the way in helping us to explore the essence of what lies within us. One of my favorite sayings comes from "spiritual great" Dolly Parton (I like to call her the Socrates from Tennessee), who said, "Find out who you really are, then go do it on purpose." The art of self-study allows us not only to *learn* who we are but intentionally *be* who we really are.

During a particularly difficult time in my

mid-teens, a good family friend presented me with a gold disk that says "Know thy self, and ye shall know the mystery." It has helped me every day of my life. Little did I realize that "know thy self" was really a tiger in disguise. With one leap, it bit into my heart, never to let go. My life has been a journey to know myself, and along the way, learn about the great mysteries of life.

RELAXATION
(Savasana)

In order to journey inward—and also to effectively practice the postures of yoga—we need to be able to relax both our bodies and our minds. When we consciously relax body and mind, they are temporarily relieved of their performing duties. The muscles can let go, and the mind can go into neutral gear for a while. Relaxation can ease you into sleep, help manage stress, quiet your mind, reconnect you to contentment, and much, much more. In fact, most of the other "tools" we've packed for this journey so far are greatly enhanced by relaxation.

There are many relaxation techniques used in our modern times, and all are valuable. I've guided students through relaxation thousands of times and always find the inner journey to be satisfying, different, and fascinating. It is interesting to note that possibly the first relaxation technique came from India and was written in the *Yoga sutra* hundreds of years ago by Patanjali. It is called *pratyahara* (withdrawal of the senses).

Throughout this book, I will guide your relaxation journey through the layers of your multidimensional Self. Specific relaxation exercises will be given, and soon you'll be able to tap into these techniques anytime, whenever you need them. Relaxation may become one of your favorite things in your suitcase.

MEDITATION
(Dhyana)

When I first tried meditation, the experience was borderline painful, both physically and mentally. The spartan instructions given to me were, "Sit on a cushion, legs in Half Lotus Pose. Close your eyes, watch your breath; don't think or move for the next 30 minutes."

Well, folks, it was hard! The first 5 minutes were fine. Then my knees and back ached. My ankles burned. Soon my legs went to sleep. Everything that could itch did. All my mind could do was silently yell, "Get me out of here!" I'm sure most of you can imagine having the same reaction.

I can honestly say I'm glad I've stuck with it. The payoff is not how great you feel during meditation. It is how you feel for the rest of the day—clear and heart-centered. Similar to relaxation, meditation provides a pathway for us to connect with our concentration, our detachment, and all the other elements we are taking with us on this journey.

Meditation may sound off-the-wall or New Age to you, but it's actually very *old* age. It's one of the oldest disciplines, practiced by wise people in virtually every part of the world. I can imagine many people thinking, "I'll try yoga, but meditation—no way!" Let me reassure you it's not New Age. It may have spiritual connotations, but it's not connected exclusively with any religion. In fact, almost every religion has a meditation component to it.

There are almost as many systems of meditation as there are people who ask, "How do I meditate?" Later in this book, I'm going to give you some specific techniques to guide you into your own version of meditation. Your goal will be to find what works for you and what doesn't. Most important, you'll decide for yourself if meditation is something you want to continue carrying with you on this journey toward your Self.

READY FOR THE JOURNEY

Until now, I've been giving you introductions to yoga concepts. I hope you're getting a feel for the journey of discovery we're going to take together. The next five sections are going to go deeply into each kosha individually, and I'll begin teaching you stretches, meditations, breathing techniques, and other aspects of yoga that work wonderfully for those of us in the midday of life. Ready to travel deeper? Let's go.

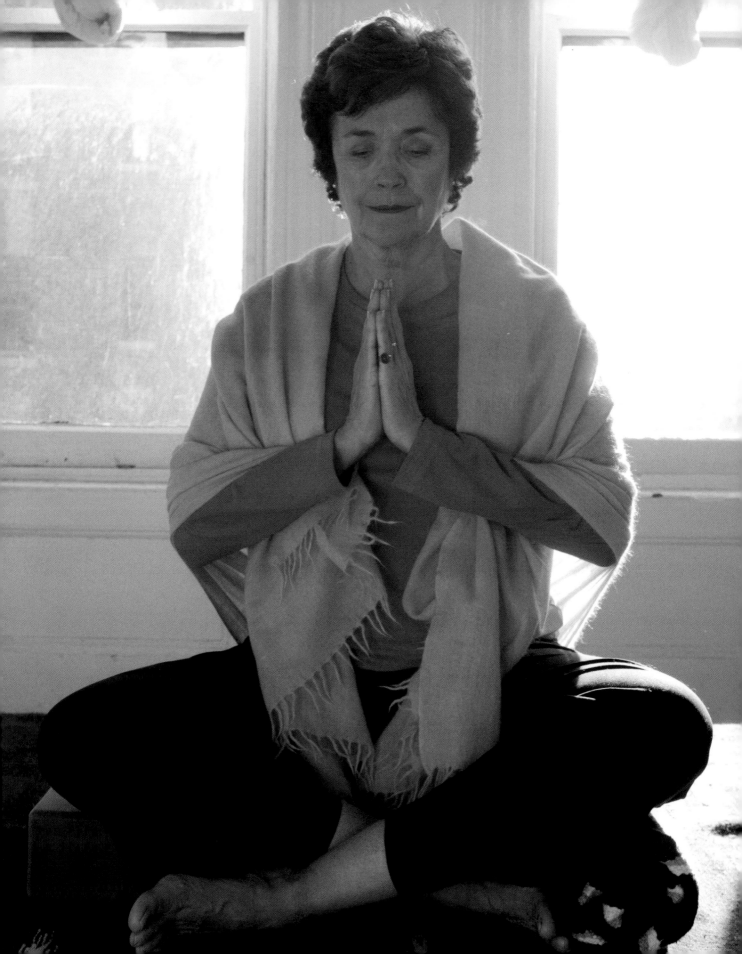

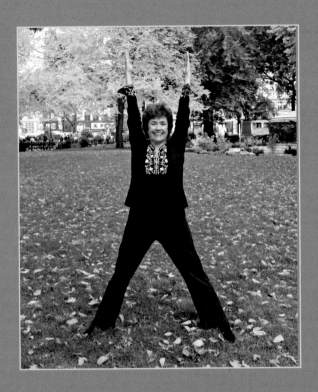

PART THREE

ANNA-MAYA-KOSHA

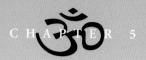

CHAPTER 5

YOUR PHYSICAL BODY

The Sanskrit name for the sheath known as the physical body is *anna-maya-kosha*, also known as the "gross" or "food" body. In today's world, it seems a bit strange to use the word "gross" when describing our body. I'm sure ancient yogis did not use it as my children might: "Oh, Mom, are you really going to eat that oyster? *Gross!*" Our physical body is only gross because we can touch and see it. The food you ate yesterday becomes the hair and teeth of tomorrow. This body is made up of bone, muscle, connecting tissue, organs, and blood, all wrapped neatly in skin, decorated with nails, eyelashes, and hair. Amazing!

Amazing though it is, our physical body is stressed and affected by many things: how we sit or stand, temperature changes, repetitive movements, what we eat and drink, and what we are thinking.

It is typical of all of us to ignore our body's discomforts until messages, which start as a whisper, become the cosmic bellow: "Hello? Anybody home?" You need to pay attention to how you feel because being separated from those messages emanating from our brain is a form of stress.

Sometimes these nonverbal messages come in the form of feelings or pictures. Recognizing them could be as simple as being aware of the whereabouts of your right hand and your left hand. Think for a moment about where you feel stress in your body and what words describe it: "knot in the gut," "uptight," "shouldering responsibilities," "butterflies in the stomach," "pain in the neck"—they all represent places on your body.

I've asked this question of yoga students all over the world. During one trip to Russia I asked, "Where do you feel stress?" Inevitably, someone said in Russian, "A pain in the butt!" There was laughter as heads nodded in understanding. I assured my Russian students that there's a word for hemorrhoids in all languages, and the problems that cause them are just as universal: too much pushing in all aspects of our stress-filled lives and inattention to sufficient water and appropriate foods needed to relieve the problem.

I will help you to increase your body awareness through what I call a yin approach to yoga asanas, relaxation, and breathing, which I'll explain in chapter 8. This is an important part of the healing journey. As you comfortably and enjoyably increase your body awareness—listening to the messages, including those of tension and stress—you'll begin cultivating the foundation for *Savasana* in the art of relaxation. The yin stretches and warmups, plus yoga movements that are well coordinated with breathing and relaxation, will remove stiffness and tension from the body. They restore vitality, stamina, and strength; improve balance and coordination; and increase the efficiency of body processes such as digestion, elimination, and detoxification.

At midlife especially, we need and appreciate a conscious, intelligent, nonmechanical approach to exercise—the yin approach—that involves the whole person . . . body, mind, and spirit.

A man has many skins in himself,
Covering the depths of his heart.
Man knows so many things;
He does not know himself.
Why, thirty or forty skins or hides,
Just like an ox's or a bear,
So thick and hard,
Cover the soul.
Go into your own ground
And learn to know yourself there.
—Meister Eckhart (1260–1328)

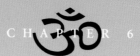
WARMUPS ARE NOT WIMPY!

Because many people think of yoga as simply a type of stretching, it doesn't occur to them that they'd benefit from warming up before starting a yoga practice. I like to teach my students several techniques of warming up. Those of us in the midday of life particularly benefit from this!

As you enter the first moments of a yoga practice, you will probably want a brief transition time. Try letting the business of the outer world go with the short relaxation shown opposite.

After your transition, you are ready to move into some form of warming up, preparing for the asanas. There are no hard and fast rules for warmups, but I have designed several that work for me. Creative warmups are designed to enhance flexibility, increase circulation, loosen muscular connecting tissue, and release tension.

DYNAMIC MOVEMENT

Some postures are done dynamically. This just means that instead of holding a pose in a static or still position, we add movement to the posture, warming up the big muscles of the body quickly and enjoyably. Begin with simple forward bends and easy sequences that open and fold and unfold the body again and again.

Some examples of the postures that can be done dynamically to warm up are:

▹ Standing Forward Bends (page 70)
▹ Thunderbolt Pose (page 152)
▹ Ring the Gong (page 55)
▹ Crescent Moon (page 179)
▹ Standing Inchworm (page 60)

Remember, there are no absolute rules for this warmup time. You are assisting muscle and fascia to release in creative, nonaggressive ways that cool, focus, and calm, with occasional flashes of heat.

At the end of your warmup, you should feel more alert, coordinated, physically warm, and comfortable in your skin. Your breathing will

LETTING GO

- Lie down on your mat. Close your eyes and daydream of a clear mountain stream. Hear it rush by . . . imagine you are sitting on the bank . . . legs dangling in the cool waters.
- Inhale . . . make a tight fist . . . feel the tension . . . hold it . . . then exhale. Let it flow . . . the tensions, worries, and cares of your day dissolve into the water.
- Inhale . . . tighten your legs, stretch your toes gently . . . let the tension build.
- Exhaling, let the tensions from your legs and arms dissolve into the water. Feel the warm sun on your skin . . . your mind peacefully centered on the beauty of the moment. Tensions of the day have passed and are forgotten . . . only this relaxing moment remains.
- Rest quietly in this pleasant state for a minute or two longer.

have deepened, and your eyesight should sharpen. And best of all, you will not feel tired.

Try 10 minutes of warmups to start your day or begin your yoga practice. You can also do 3 minutes of well-thought-out warmups to prepare your body for a particular asana (posture).

Your body will respond more positively if you do your warmup stretches in a certain sequence.

Try to work in this order:

- Neck, upper back, then lower back
- The sides of your body
- Arms before chest
- Seat muscles before groin
- Calves before hamstrings
- Shins before thighs

SELF-MASSAGE

Sometimes I use self-massage, such as tapping or thumping the hamstring or shoulder muscle with a cupped hand or gently closed fist. Tapping muscle fibers helps them to "warm up" or release their tightness. Try this now and see for yourself.

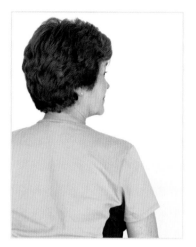

- Sit tall in your chair, with your shoulders directly above your hips. With awareness, look over your right shoulder. Come to a natural stopping point. Find a spot on the wall, and remember it. Return your head to center.

- Now bring your left arm across your chest and with a cupped hand, firmly tap your right shoulder for 15 to 30 taps. Tap . . . tap . . . tap . . .

- Again slowly look over your right shoulder. Remember your stopping point in the first step? Have you gone further? Have you increased your range of motion just a little? Chances are you are saying yes. Now, repeat this tapping warmup on the other shoulder.

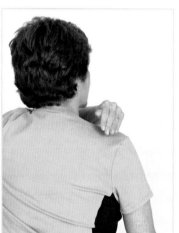

ROLLING AROUND

Rolling around on the floor could be considered another form of warming up. I ask students to mind-fully roll on the floor or on a ball, using their body weight as an overall massage to purposefully soften the body's connective tissue, specifically fascia.

Most of us are familiar with terms like joints, ligaments, cartilage, and muscle, but the subject of fascia and maintaining its midlife health is just coming into its own.

FUN WITH FASCIA

For a sometimes dramatic and easily done demonstration of how warming up and working one small body part can affect the functioning of the whole, start at the soles of your feet. This sole consists of thick fascia layers. Like the sole of your shoe, it protects your foot.

BENEFITS: *This self-massage can be used to keep your feet feeling great. It is also interesting to do the same three steps with Downward-Facing Dog (see page 149) as the posture, measuring where the heels touch the floor. The results can be quite dramatic.*

- First, do this simple test, a forward bend. No big deal—just sit on the floor with your legs extended in front of you, knees straight. Lean forward, extend your arms, and note the final resting position of your hands on the floor. Hold, with your eyes closed, and observe how it feels along the back and sides of your body. Hold for 10 breaths, you and your witness taking mental notes.

- Return to sitting up. Now I'd like you to roll a golf ball or tennis ball deeply into the bottom of one foot only. Go slowly behind and on top of your toes, ball, arch, and the edges of your heel. Be thorough rather than fast and vigorous. Keep it up for 2 to 3 minutes, covering the whole territory of the foot.

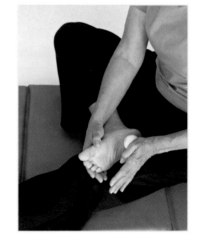

- Now repeat the forward bend again. Go slowly, folding forward. Close your eyes and feel the difference in one side compared with the other. Note your final hand position. Take your time. Pay attention to what you are feeling.

YIN TIP: *Massaging the fascia aids in releasing it. This in turn helps release tissue throughout the leg and back. Get up and walk around. Feel the difference in one foot compared with the other. Be sure to do these same steps on the opposite foot.*

FASCINATING FASCIA FACTS

- Fascia is like a Saran Wrap body bag made of gel. It surrounds and holds your body together—every muscle, organ, blood vessel.
- Fascia facilitates every movement of your body. It enables your muscles to move over and around organs without friction or resistance.
- It allows individual muscles to lengthen and shorten with ease.
- Fascia consistency changes with aging. It begins to lose resiliency in our late 20s and will continue to contract every 7 to 10 years thereafter.
- Age, injury, stress, toxins, inactivity, and excessive activity affect fascia. It is thought that even powerful emotions and thoughts can possibly burrow deeply into fascia.
- Fascia does not respond well to brief, rhythmical stretches the way muscles do.
- It is tough and fibrous and best pulled (warmed up) slowly, like taffy.
- Fascia accelerates its natural contracting process when you are ill or injured.

Still having trouble picturing fascia? Imagine pulling on a rubber dishwashing glove. Then pull a woolen glove over it. The rubber glove is the fascia; the woolen glove is muscle.

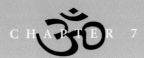

CHAPTER 7

SAVASANA: THE ART OF RELAXATION

"WELCOME ALL THAT COMES TO YOU THIS DAY, AND FEEL WELCOMED BY IT."

—*Jean Klein*

Relaxation pose is known as Savasana, usually translated as "Corpse Pose." I always felt squeamish about calling it Corpse on national television. For years I've called relaxation by its tame, second name, Sponge Pose. Why would anyone desire to practice being a corpse? It has taken a while for me to understand that the label "corpse" is very appropriate. In Savasana, we lie on our back, eyes closed, completely still. Outwardly, we look dead to the world. But inwardly, the witness is alive and awake, monitoring all the layers of body-mind-spirit.

Practicing guided relaxation in Sponge Pose, under the watchful eye of your witness, reveals the hidden inner spaces of the body. Of course, these inner spaces exist only in our imagination. But that's what imagination is for, so let's use it! With the help of the breath and the witness

watching, it is easy to calm and relax the body and look inward.

Savasana or relaxation can be done in three ways:

1. A short "let go" relaxation done as a transition from a busy day, in the beginning of a yoga session, or as a "minute vacation" between postures.
2. Yogoda dynamic relaxation, also done at the beginning of a yoga session.
3. A longer guided relaxation at the end of the session.

SHORT LET-GO RELAXATION

It is not wise to come home from your busy day and plunge directly into asana practice. The mind and body need a little time to separate from one life activity to another. Try letting the business of the outer world go with this short transitional relaxation.

- Lie down on the mat . . . close your eyes.
- Lift your arms ½ inch off the mat . . . pause . . . then let them drop . . . with a sigh.
- Lift your hips ½ inch . . . pause . . . let them flop . . . with a sigh.
- Keep your heels to the floor . . . hands on your knees . . . lift the hips and thighs . . . with a big sigh . . . Let them flop.
- Now lift your arms, hips, and thighs off mat . . . big let-go sigh . . . let go. All the phone calls, rushing around, car pools, details of life . . . mentally let them go. Finish with one last open-mouth, deep, let-go sigh . . . this time really mean it. Rest quietly in a "minute vacation."

YOGODA DYNAMIC RELAXATION OF THE PHYSICAL BODY

BENEFITS: *This relaxation exercise places dynamic tension at different times on arms, legs, and the whole body. It deeply relaxes the muscles, and vitality can be felt almost immediately.*

CAUTION: *Please omit yogoda if you have high blood pressure and/or heart challenges.*

- Lie down on your well-padded surface. (My Lili-Pad yoga mat is perfect.) Your feet are shoulder-width apart and your arms lie a few inches away from the sides of your body, palms up. Tuck your shoulder blades in toward your spine; make sure they're not bunched up toward your ears.
- With your eyes closed, focus your attention on your legs. Now cross your ankles. Breathe deeply in . . . holding the breath . . . tighten your legs by gently trying to pull your ankles apart. Hold for 3 seconds . . . then *exhale.* Uncross your ankles . . . let your legs flop apart. Pause . . . feel the sensation within your legs.
- Now repeat the sequence, crossing your ankles in the opposite direction. Then uncross your ankles . . . let your legs flop apart. Pause . . . feel the sensation within your legs.
- Focus on your arms . . . breathe in . . . stretch your arms . . . lift them up an inch . . . open your fingers like a star . . . hold the breath and count to 3 . . . now exhale completely. Arms drop . . . feel the sensation that follows within your arms. Pause . . . let your whole body get heavy.
- Now, be aware of all separate parts of your body. Then . . . inhale through your nose, deep breath in . . . tighten and *tense* your whole body all at once. Make a good prune face . . . squeeze your eyes, your mouth, your cheeks together. Tighten your arms . . . shoulders . . . legs. Mild tension at first . . . hold for 3 seconds . . . release . . . relax. Enjoy the sensations that follow . . . feel your body float.
- The tension should begin mildly, progressing to medium, then to medium high. Do the dy-

namic tension three times, enjoying a short relaxation between each tensing.

LONGER RELAXATION

Longer relaxation is always done at the end of a yoga session, after warmups and asanas. But why do you need relaxation after practicing mindful stretches? It helps you "seal" your yoga practice within your body and mind. It helps you take the inspiration of yoga into the rest of your day. It is very different than falling asleep in front of your television or pumping iron at the gym. It is setting aside at least 5 to 10 minutes at the end of your yoga session to consciously relax your body. "Conscious" relaxation might sound a bit New Agey, but it's very practical. Your witness is present, alert and aware, detached and serene, observing the body release surface tensions and, sometimes, deeply layered physical and emotional stress. In this state of relaxation, the body and mind become refreshed, recharged, and rejuvenated. It is a condition of deep, quiet rest.

Remember, to rest is to heal. Physiologically, relaxation is characterized by a slower heart rate, lower blood pressure and rate of breathing, and slower brain-wave patterns.

The Four Steps of Deep Relaxation

There are four aspects of relaxation. The first is to *focus* your attention like a searchlight on different parts of your body. Second is to *suggest*, using your inner talking to your advantage, rather than letting it use you with mindless chatter. The third aspect is to *pause* or wait. This is a moment to sharpen your inner awareness. The fourth is to *feel* the sensations, what's going on inside your body. This is not a moment to judge or evaluate. It is a moment to feel. When a body part relaxes, there are usually pleasant feelings. Stay attentive to these feelings! Today you are different than you were yesterday. That's why this practice is always interesting and fun.

Remember: Focus. Suggest. Pause. Feel.

Please go over, again and again, the following steps to relaxation. Relaxation thrives on repetition. It is that important and that interesting. The components—focus, suggest, pause, feel—will stay the same each time you practice, but your experience of the results will change each time you practice them. Practice different segments often, any time of day. The four steps simplify the art of relaxation. Your evaluating mind can move aside and allow the witness observer to awaken and go ever deeper into the Self.

Now, let's set the stage for relaxation. Turn off your cell phone, kick off your shoes, loosen your waistband. Sit in a comfortable chair or lie down. I hope your room is comfortably warm and your door is closed. Tell your family and your pets that this is your special time to relax. *Do not disturb.*

I know it can be hard in a small apartment or house—or one with small children—to designate a place for your hatha and relaxation practice. If possible, keep handy two blankets, two pillows, an eye pillow or washcloth, a CD or cassette player, and instructional relaxation CDs and tapes.

I also know this is difficult to do while you read the following words. You might enjoy listening to a CD from the NaturalJourneys.com Discover series, or reading this text and recording your own voice, pausing at the ellipses. Play it back for deep relaxation. Remember, I am merely your guide. You and you alone have the final authority and right to decide what you will and will not do. This is your precious time of relaxation, a time to let your day go.

LONG RELAXATION EXERCISE (MAHA SAVASANA)

The following maha (long) relaxation takes about 5 minutes. This relaxation is about feeling. Try pausing to feel the relaxation inside each limb. Sometimes you have to wait a breath or two for the feelings to come, so take your time. This enjoyable relaxation releases muscle tension, quiets the mind, and reduces fatigue. When the eyes are still, thinking slows down.

- Begin by sitting on your well-padded surface. (Again, my Lili-Pad yoga mat is perfect.) Place a pillow beneath your knees. This will allow your back to sink deeper into your mat. Feet should be shoulder-width apart. Cover yourself with a blanket, as body temperature cools with deep relaxation.

- Lower your back to the mat. Place the second pillow beneath your head if you want (most folks do). Adjust the angle of your chin by sliding the back of your head upward ¼ inch. This will lower your chin slightly. Place an eye pillow or cloth across your eyes, keeping them in total darkness, allowing them to be still.

- Take a few long, slow breaths, emphasizing the long exhale.

- Bring awareness to your right leg, from your toes to your hip. Roll the leg from side to side, then feel the leg get heavy.

- Focus on your left leg. Roll it from side to side, without disturbing the rest of your body. Pause. Feel the left leg get heavy.

- Focus on your right arm, shoulder to elbow. Pause. Then focus on your right hand. Feel the sensations in your right hand: Warm? Cool? Tingly?

- Focus on your left arm: shoulder, elbow, wrist, hand. Pause. Feel the sensations within your hand. Take your time. Wait for the feelings to come.

- Focus on your hips and seat muscle. Feel both sides of your seat muscle equally. Exhale. Feel the hips get heavy, and the muscles soften. Become aware of the floor supporting them.

- Bring your awareness to your chest and lungs. Feel your inhale as the chest and lungs expand. Exhale. Feel your chest, lungs, and heart relaxing . . . melting. Your breath is smooth and easy.

- Focus on your neck. Gently, without disturbing your torso, inhale and roll your head

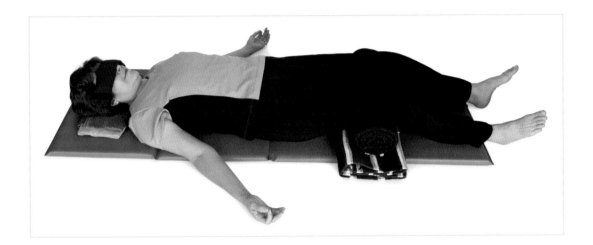

left. Pause. Exhaling, roll your head to the right, then back to center. Bring your chin down slightly toward your chest. Allow your head to find its center naturally. Pause.

- Scan your face. Soften the little lines of the forehead. Feel where your eyelids touch. Feel the length of your lips. Unlock your jaw muscle . . . feel it soften.

- Observe your whole body, heavy, spacious, free from tightness or muscle tension. And now

rest . . . in this timeless moment.

- To come out of relaxation . . . without moving . . . *feel* your whole body . . . then slowly raise your arms over your head and give your body a wonderful head-to-toe stretch. Roll over onto your right side, knees to your chest. Pause . . . ask yourself, what stress can I leave here on the mat? Slowly . . . come up to a seated position. Open your eyes. Have a great day!

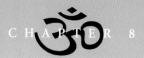

CHAPTER 8

THE YIN APPROACH

Why is it that the midlife body becomes stiff and tight? One reason is that in our late 20s, muscle and connective tissue become less resilient and will continue to lose flexibility as we age. Life's stress, wear-and-tear injuries, and inactivity leave their mark in the muscles and soft tissue. The older we get, the more "creaky" we might feel. Can a middle-aged body return to a graceful, fluid suppleness? My answer is an unqualified *yes!* But how? This is the focus of the yin approach to warming up, stretching, and asanas.

THE YOGA MIRACLE

I enjoy being a student in other people's yoga classes, especially those taught by master yoga teacher Angela Farmer. I was in one such class when I made a discovery. I was doing a Traditional Seated Forward Bend, legs extended, torso folded over thighs. My partner knelt behind me and applied gentle pressure to my lower back to help me lengthen my spine and go further into the stretch. But I found if I arched my back just a little, pushed my spine into her hands (the opposite direction of Forward Bend), held the resistance for a few seconds, relaxed, and then redid the posture, I could comfortably slide even further and deeper into the pose.

In effect, I had tightened my muscle just before relaxing it for the stretch. I wondered if this concept could be applied to other yoga postures, helping me to get a better stretch. Over the years, I experimented in my own practice and found that these small moves could be effective in many other yoga poses.

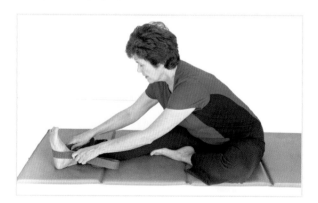

Later I came across a technique called PNF, which stands for proprioceptive neuromuscular facilitation. Scientific research supports the PNF phenomenon, but Larry Payne (coauthor of *Yoga for Dummies*) refers to it as the "yoga miracle." It's miraculous because the results are instant, painless, and amazing! It is widely used by athletes and trainers, and different variations exist, but the way I incorporate it into most yoga routines is unique. The basic technique involves alternating isometric muscle contraction and passive stretching. Before stretching a muscle, you tighten it and push against a fixed object—a partner, your own hand, a belt, the floor, or a wall. The subsequent stretch becomes longer, deeper, and far more comfortable than holding the limb in a static stretch. (See Appendix A to learn about the yoga belt and other props.)

For some years, I've adapted this way of stretching to my own middle-aged body and for those who take classes from me. I developed the "three Rs"—Resist, Relax, and Restretch. I always love seeing students' amazement at the improvement in their own flexibility. While other yoga teachers mention the PNF phenomenon and occasionally tell their students about it, I've made it an integral part of the way I teach yoga. No one else teaches yoga quite the same way. Today I call it a yin approach to stretching (not to be confused with yin yoga, in which poses are held for several minutes).

The concepts of yin and yang are from the Taoist tradition. If something is yin, it can be de-scribed as cool, calm, inward, and focused, like a stretching posture in yoga. The concept of yang is moving, heated, excited, intense, like a strength posture. Most postures and well-balanced yoga classes have both a yin and yang component. Like a new piece added to a puzzle, I enjoy doing a yin stretch, balanced with yang strength, in almost all yoga postures. It makes my middle-aged muscles feel safer, more comfortable, and complete while in the pose. I find this approach to be effective for the beginner as well as the experienced student of hatha yoga.

The Yin Approach to Stretching

To get the feel of the yin approach to stretching, practice the following exercise.

STEP ONE

Lie on your back, both knees bent, feet flat on the floor. Extend your right leg up to the ceiling

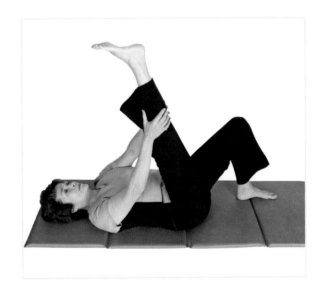

as straight as possible. Interlock your hands around your right calf, or behind the back of your knee or thigh (see photo below). If you prefer, you can use a belt over the sole of your foot. Without bouncing or causing pain, pull your leg toward your head, keeping your knee straight.

Hold statically for six to eight breaths. Look at your toes. Notice how far your leg has lengthened against a spot on the ceiling, and make a mental note.

Release your leg and repeat on the opposite side, then release.

STEP TWO, THE THREE RS

RESIST: Again, extend your right leg up to the ceiling as straight as possible. Place both hands around the back of your thigh, one hand over the other (or loop the belt over the sole of your foot, and reach up and hold on to the belt, one hand on either side of your foot). Be sure your

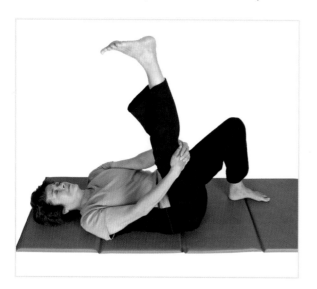

leg is not pressed in close to your chest. Your elbows are almost straight, and your lower leg is passive. Push your thigh into your hand, and with your hand, press back into your thigh. If you're using the belt, push your leg upward as you gently pull the belt toward you to create resistance. This is not red-faced resistance; it is a gentle, firm, steady, no-bounce contraction of muscles. Hold for 8 seconds, breathing comfortably behind the resistance.

RELAX: After resistance is over, you now exhale and Relax, still holding your thigh. Breathe in, then with a long exhale, feel the muscles you've just used for the resistance soften. Relax your arms. Let your abdomen and leg go limp. Close your eyes and notice the warm and tingly relaxation feeling. Without moving and still holding your leg, pause for a moment.

RESTRETCH: Repeat the same stretch as in step one. Go very, very slowly. Take your time. Your high awareness is needed as you feel the fibers of your hamstrings lengthen without any pain. Extend your leg toward the ceiling and, moving in increments, gently pull it in the direction of your right shoulder, without bending your knee. Do not hold your breath—breathing is shallow and comfortable. Now, take another peek at your toes. Notice that your hamstrings have lengthened even more! Voilà—the miracle! Hold for 30 seconds (10 breaths), and repeat on the opposite leg.

Sometimes, if I feel especially stiff, I spend a few minutes stretching using the three Rs. I like to repeat each three-R sequence a few times, but I've found that no significant further range of motion can be achieved beyond three repetitions.

Many times a new middle-aged student of the yin approach will experience a breakthrough if a tight muscle is suddenly able to move into a new range of motion. What a moment! But don't be discouraged if you feel tightening up again within minutes. Improvement is cumulative. My students report that a significant lengthening remains and is noticeable in the next session.

I used to think I had to stretch every day in order to become and keep flexible. Today, I've found that the middle-aged student who really gets the hang of this yin way of stretching can do it two or three times a week and be more flexible than those who statically stretch (the "old" way) each and every day.

Later chapters will include a yoga plan with instructions for 20 postures and their yin components.

Guidelines for Using the Three Rs Effectively

▶ In all of yoga, form and alignment are all-important. The photos and descriptions are there to illustrate the *form* of the three Rs when used within a stretch, warmup, and some asanas.

▶ Hold the final Restretch position for the recommended time. If you hold longer, you will overdo the stretch, which can cause injuries. The length of time to hold in the final position will be expressed in breaths: one breath equals an inhale and exhale. Ten breaths equal about 30 seconds. Large muscles are held for a longer time; short muscles, a shorter time.

▶ When using the three Rs, do not let the limb that is being contracted move at all. Any movement, like bouncing the limb, reduces the final stretch, often significantly.

▶ When you do the Resistance, do not push too hard. This is not a struggle. Remember, keep cool, calm, and focused.

▶ Relax, the second R . . . You know how to relax. Let your whole body go limp. Feel it happen and remember to exhale.

▶ Give some thought to the idea that if you are using the three Rs to stretch a muscle or limb, it is out of its normal range of motion. It is only sensible, and also feels good, safe, and nurturing, to use other muscles to help return your stretched limb back to its starting position.

▶ Use the three Rs to help you locate muscles in your body. You don't have to know a particular muscle's name. However, performing a gentle contraction brings that area into your awareness and will enhance your stretching efforts considerably.

▶ The three Rs are a creative way to listen to your body. Listening to your body is a life-long journey. You can use the three Rs throughout all the seasons of your life.

You will get a fabulous all-over body stretch just doing these yin warmups by themselves. These moves are less strict in form and alignment and will put large and small muscles plus connecting tissue through many ranges of motion that conventional asanas do not. Using them in combination with asanas, however, you will safely go deeper and get more out of each posture.

Yin Warmups for Upper Body

Rolling around on a soft ball wakes up your tired neck and shoulders. These nice side-to-side motions invite you to get "into your own skin," especially in the hard-to-reach area between your shoulder blades and upper neck. With the slow and gentle rolling, your body weight against the ball warms and softens fascia.

I use a soft to medium-soft (which I prefer) rubber ball of medium size, which can be found in the children's section of your local department store.

CAUTION: If the ball hurts your neck, do these moves without a ball. Do not do this rolling if you have arthritis or bone-density issues.

UPPER NECK CURVE

- Lie on a mat on your back, with your neck in neutral position. Then bend your knees and rest your head comfortably on the ball, supporting the curve of your neck. Your shoulders are off the mat.

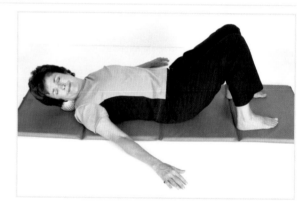

- Slowly roll your head from side to side, stretching your neck muscles in a way that's enjoyable. Five times each side . . . breathing easily . . . relax jaw muscles.

- Now bring your chin to your chest to lengthen the back of your neck muscles. This should feel good on your neck. Then, slowly raise your chin toward the ceiling. Move back and forth five times. Inhale as you raise your chin; exhale as you lower it.

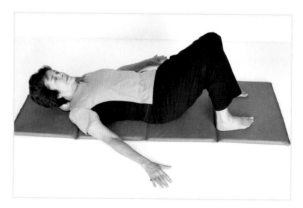

SHOULDER ROLL

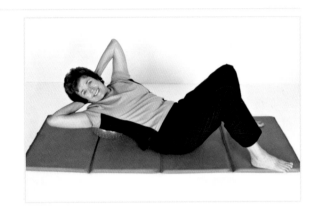

- After doing the Upper Neck Curve, move the ball down between your shoulder blades, keeping your shoulders off the mat. Clasp your hands behind the base of your neck for support. Your weight is now on your sacrum (the base of your spine) and seat muscles. Your lower back is long and comfortable. Your hands comfortably support your upper neck. There is space between your chin and chest.

- Now, roll from side to side over your shoulder blades five or six times. Move slowly with this natural twisting motion. Inhale on one side, exhale on the other side.

LOW BACK ROLLING

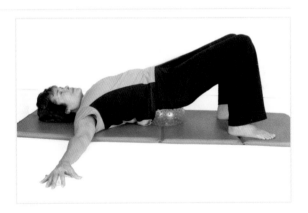

- If you want to get a little wild, place the ball beneath your sacrum and hips. Keep your arms and feet on the mat for balance. Now, roll from side to side, from hip to hip . . . then tailbone to waist, all different directions.

  YIN TIP: *Remember to stay in your comfort zone. Even though this is easy and fun, too much rolling can make you a little sore.*

- Variation: Keep the ball beneath your hips and raise your feet to the ceiling, then roll from side to side. Fun!

STARGAZING SITUP

This is your classic gym "situp" with interesting and effective tweaks to strengthen the upper abs, insides of legs (adductors), the neck, and shoulders.

- Lie on your back, knees bent and feet on the floor, hip-width apart. Turn your toes in (as though pigeon-toed) and press your knees together. Your arms assume the stargazing position: Spread your palms on the back of your head, fingers interlocked, elbows wide. Imagine you are on a grassy slope, looking up into the dark night sky.

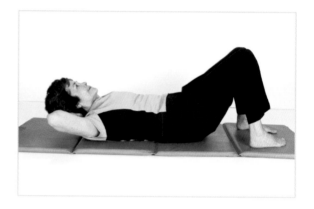

- Exhaling, press your knees firmly, using your core muscles behind your navel. Tilt the front of your pelvis toward your navel, keeping your hips on the mat, and slowly sit up halfway.

  YIN TIP: *Keep your elbows wide in the stargazing position. Support your head. Look toward the night sky. Don't yank your head up with your arms. Come up by contracting your abdominals.*

- Inhaling, roll down slowly. Repeat the situp six to eight times.

NECK TILT I

BENEFITS: *I carry a great deal of tension in my neck and shoulders. I love this exercise series and can feel improvement immediately. These simple, effective moves can be done anytime, anywhere, such as during an hourly break from the computer. The whole sequence takes only 4 minutes and is a great way to begin your warmup session.*

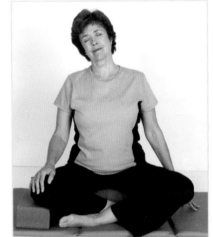

- Sit tall with your shoulders down. Use props if needed, such as a block under the knee or a pillow under the seat. Tilt your head to the right side. Rather than bringing your ear to shoulder, consciously extend and elongate your neck into the space to your right. The opposite shoulder and side of the neck will lengthen as well. Hold for three breaths. Repeat on the other side.

NECK TILT II

BENEFITS: *Stretching the neck muscles has an immediate effect on your state of mind. Lengthening the larger muscles defuses stress held in the body and helps the whole body to relax. Lengthening and stretching small neck muscles will help quiet the mind and bring on a sense of well-being. This can also help prevent tension headaches.*

- Do Neck Tilt I, but use the three Rs. Reach your right hand up above your left ear. Use this hand as a little wall. Press your head gently into your hand, and your hand into your head. Resist for three breaths, without moving. Stop pushing, Relax, and breathe in. Exhale. Now Restretch. Softly use your hand to guide your head a little further into the space to the right. Lower your hand and hold for two or three breaths. Repeat on the opposite shoulder. Observe which side is tighter.

CHIN TO CHEST

This is a nice stretch to prepare your neck for Half Shoulderstand (page 193) and Bridge Pose (page 156).

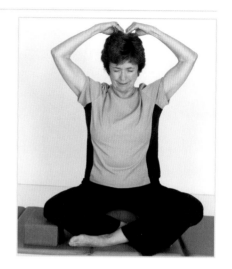

- Sit tall and comfortably in a chair or on the floor with your legs folded. (If you're on the floor, sit on a cushion to help your spine tip slightly forward.) Now slowly lower your chin. Feel the weight of your head as the back of your neck and shoulders stretch. Rest in the stretch for two or three breaths, then lift your chin and return your head to neutral position.

- Then, still sitting tall, drop your chin halfway to your chest. Reach up with your hands and place a few fingers on the highest part of your head. Now do the three Rs.

- Resist: Gently press your skull back into your fingers while your fingers gently press into your skull. Do not move your head during the resistance. Count to three. Relax, breathe in. Carefully and slowly Restretch. Hold your head like a bowling ball. Exhale, relax, and feel your neck muscles lengthen. Drop your head forward, chin moving closer to your chest. Rest in the stretch for two or three breaths. Return your head back to neutral position.

SINGING SNAKE

BENEFITS: *The neck holds a valuable source of information about yourself. Neck muscles react strongly to stress. The alignment of your neck, jaw, shoulders, and head silently says a great deal to the world about what you are really thinking and feeling. I call this Singing Snake because it can be used as a variation of Cobra Pose. After the Chin to Chest, there is a natural cue from within to go in the opposite direction, but many people find dropping the head back uncomfortable. Try Singing Snake in the following way, which should be more comfortable.*

- Sitting tall, breathe in with a slack jaw, and relax your body. Exhale. Then open your mouth as wide as possible. With your mouth open, slowly tilt your head back, then tilt your neck back as well. Relax your shoulders. This should feel more comfortable than if you had just tipped your head back.

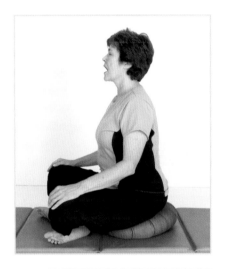

- Once your head is tilted all the way back, very slowly close your teeth and lips. When you close your teeth in this extended position, you are supported by the powerful clenching jaw muscles in the front of your neck. Return your head into neutral position. Then slowly and enjoyably lower your chin to your chest to relax the muscles at the back of your neck.

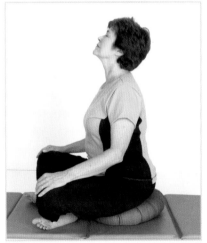

Chest Expander

BENEFITS: *Chest Expander can be done standing, kneeling, or seated in a chair, with or without a partner (see page 202). This stretch breaks up muscle tension and stress carried within the muscles of your torso. It improves posture and breathing, and can be done in business clothes. Take a time-out from the computer and do the Chest Expander on a coffee break. It energizes and clears the brain. It's tops on my list of un-wimpy warmups!*

PART ONE

- Begin by rolling each shoulder in both directions in slow circles—three to six times each way for each shoulder. Then stand, your hands behind you, palms facing your seat muscles, clasping a belt. (See Appendix A for information on the yoga belt.) Separate your hands about 4 inches more if this bothers your elbows. Note that a partner can be helpful with this warmup, as you can see me helping Kevin in the photo.

- Standing tall, roll your shoulders back and down. Straighten your elbows, lifting your arms upward, holding on to your belt. Hold for two or three breaths, allowing your muscles to stretch. Release. You will get much more out of this warmup if you add the three Rs. After you've done part one, you're ready for part two.

PART TWO

- Create the three Rs by clasping the belt and gently pulling downward. Observe how this move causes resistance and places tension on your upper back, shoulder, and arm muscles. Do not lift your arms at this point; just pull down . . . and hold the Resistance, closing the gates of your shoulders.

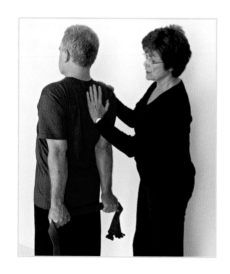

- Now Relax and Restretch . . . Stand tall and again pull down first . . . then holding the belt, lift both arms up . . . maybe go a little higher . . . lift up your heart . . . breathe in . . . chest lifts . . . tailbone is down . . . keep "heart eyes" open as you exhale . . . hold for two or three breaths. Lower your arms and release the belt . . . stand with your eyes closed . . . observe feelings of lightness in your arms and torso.

CAUTION: *Do not bend or cock your wrists. In part two, lift your arms up in increments, giving muscle fibers a chance to lengthen.*

YIN TIP: *You can use the back of a piece of furniture to assist you with the three Rs. Stand with your back to a chair, clasp the belt, and place your fists on top of the chair. Roll your shoulders back and down. Create a little resistance as you gently press downward toward the floor. Hold for a few breaths, then release. Relax and Restretch, as in part one. When finished, let go of the belt. Close your eyes and imagine any weariness of the day melting off your shoulders. Enjoy the sensations.*

SACRED MOUNTAIN POSE (*TADASANA*)

Sacred Mountain Pose, or Tadasana, is the foundation of all standing poses. I include it here so you will know the correct starting position for the following standing yin warmups.

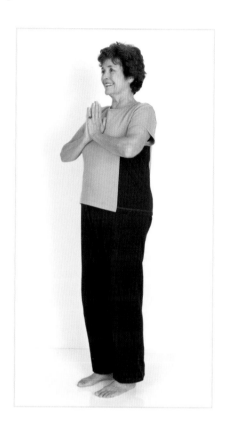

- Stand tall with your big toes touching, or feet hip-width apart. Knees are straight but not locked. To align your torso, gently point your tailbone downward and pull the core muscles behind your navel back into your spine and up. Pull your shoulders down and back. Lift up your heart.

- Place the palms of your hands together in Namaste (prayer position), then nestle the knuckles of your thumbs into the little indentation in your breastbone, called the "lake of tranquillity." Bowing the head quiets the mind.

RING THE GONG

BENEFITS: *Turning action gently stretches torso and back.*

- Stand tall in Sacred Mountain Pose. Your arms hang down heavy and relaxed, and your weight is over both feet. Swing your arms from side to side, as if you were a child. Use your torso and shoulders to help you turn gently, and let your arms follow. Keep swinging, knees bent, from side to side. Repeat six to eight times.

- Pause. Now make your hands into two soft fists, like clappers in a bell. Repeat the first step. Swing your arms around to "ring the gong" behind you, giving a little "ding" over each hip.

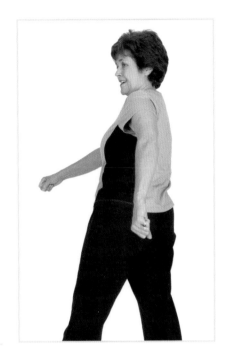

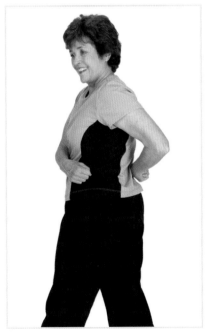

SHOULDER PREPARATION FOR GARUDA ARMS

BENEFITS: *Excellent for releasing tightness in front and back of shoulders. Great preparation for Garuda Arms. Nice warmup for long-distance swimming, or your golf or tennis swing.*

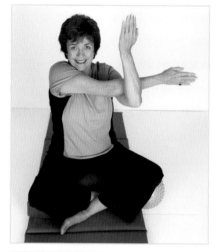

- Sit comfortably on a chair or on the floor with your legs folded. (If you're on the floor, place a cushion beneath your seat to lift your spine.) I also like to place a prop (a block or a ball) under each of my knees for support. Make sure you are comfortable and sitting up straight.

- Extend your right arm out to the side, parallel to floor. Then swing it gracefully across your body. Use the momentum to catch your right arm in the crook of your left elbow.

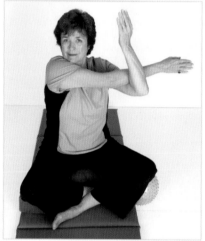

- Holding on firmly, guide your right arm up toward throat level for a better stretch. Be sure your right arm is above your chest. "Measure" and feel the natural stop of the arm stretching. Hold for three or four breaths. Now do the three Rs with your arm at throat level, pressing the straight arm away from your body while you gently Resist with the crooked elbow. Hold the resistance for 2 breaths. Relax . . . breathe in . . . exhale, Restretch. Pull the arm very, very slowly across your throat . . . hold for three to five breaths. Notice how much further your arm can stretch.

- Let the right arm go limp. Use the crook of the left elbow like a sling and slowly lower the limp right arm. Then repeat the steps on the opposite arm. To add a little heat when in the second step, hold the back of your neck with the hand of your crooked arm.

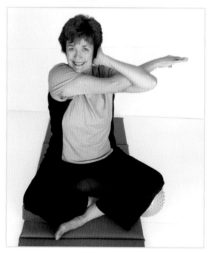

GARUDA ARMS

BENEFITS: *Enjoy the same benefits as with the Shoulder Preparation.*

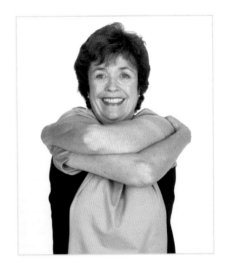

- Extend your arms out from your sides in a T position. With a big swooping motion, cross your left elbow over right elbow. Clasp your hands to shoulders. Give yourself a big hug. Hold for two or three breaths. Smile! Enjoy giving yourself a hug today.

- Now release your hands, keeping the elbows crossed. Place the backs of your hands together. If you are more flexible, put the thumb of your left hand into the palm of your right. Slowly raise both arms up and down.

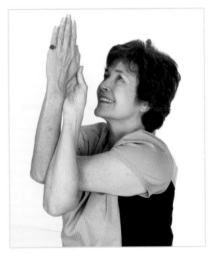

- Release your arms out from your sides to again form a T. Repeat the steps, crossing your right elbow over your left.

YIN TIP: *It is very interesting to do Garuda Arms three times, once with no yin warmup. Then do the yin warmup on both arms. On the third time, repeat Garuda Arms. The difference in ease can be amazing!*

Yin Warmups for Lower Body

Warming up your lower body can make a big difference in the comfort of your legs and hips in daily life. This is especially true during everyday walking and stairclimbing.

SHIN STRETCH WITH THREE RS

BENEFITS: *This is an excellent stretch to prevent a common problem of athletes as well as midlifers who walk on hard surfaces: shin splints. The stretching of the front shin muscle, as well as the calves and hamstrings, prepares legs for all standing postures as well as your daily walk.*

- Sit on your mat with one leg folded beside you. Your hips are level with both sit bones to the floor. This first step is a very strong stretch for everyone, so I suggest you fold a blanket and prop up the hip of the straight leg, as in the photo. Your foot on the folded leg needs to be pointing straight back behind you, not angled out. Rotating the foot out places potentially dangerous stress on the knee. To create a little more space in the folded knee, reach down and pull your calf muscle out to the side. If this stretch bothers your knees, please omit. Once in position, sit for a moment, letting the muscles stretch effortlessly. Your hands support you. Your knee is happy.

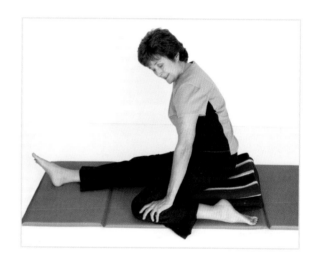

- The three Rs are done by gently pressing the toes, shinbone, and top of foot downward into the mat while you hold the knee for five to eight breaths. Relax . . . pause . . . breathe in. Consciously Relax your toes, instep, and shin muscles. Exhale . . . and Restretch. Very, very slowly lift the knee a little further. Sometimes a second brief go-round with the three Rs feels good. Hold the final Restretch for five breaths or longer. Then repeat on the opposite leg.

HAMSTRINGS SOLO, HAMSTRINGS 3-WAYS

BENEFITS: *This is a powerful way to safely stretch the hammies. Once learned, you can do it three times a week.*

- Lie on your mat on your back, with your knees bent and feet to the floor. Lift your right foot and loop the belt around the sole of your foot. Straighten your arms, reaching toward the foot. Then extend your leg toward the ceiling, with your knee slightly bent. Test the flexibility of your hamstring by pulling the leg gently toward you until you feel that first edge of resistance. (Note: My arms are straight and the belt is not wrapped around my hands.) Hold about 30 seconds.

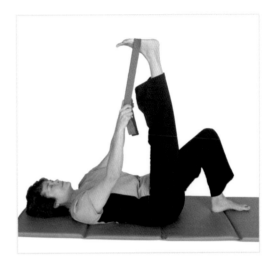

- Now bring your right leg back to its starting point. Pause . . . and begin the three Rs. Resist by pressing your foot and leg bones up into the belt, simultaneously pulling gently, steadily down with belt. *No bouncing!* Three Rs will not work as well if you bounce. Hold the Resistance . . . feel what muscles are contracting. Hold for three to five breaths . . . then Relax . . . breathe in . . . exhale and Restretch. Go very, very slowly into this last stretch and hold for about 1 minute.

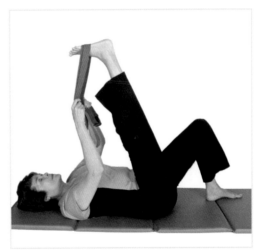

- As a variation, you can stretch the hammies three ways:
  1. Raised foot straight (as above)
  2. Raised foot turned in (pigeon-toed)
  3. Raised foot turned out (like Charlie Chaplin)

  Go through the steps for Hamstrings Solo, trying the foot in three different directions. Have fun!

STANDING INCHWORM

I use Inchworm as a way to move into Standing Forward Bend.

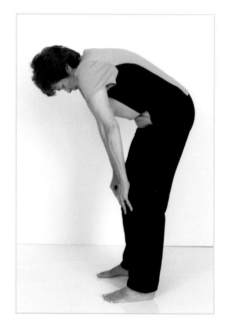

- Start by standing tall, then bring your chin to your chest. Upper body slumps forward. Now, place your hands on your thighs for support. Pressing your hands into your thighs, round your back like a cat, exhaling.

- Inhaling, go in the opposite direction, lifting your tailbone and chin. Your low back forms a little valley. Now move slowly back and forth, inhaling and exhaling, like a little inchworm making its way across a leaf.

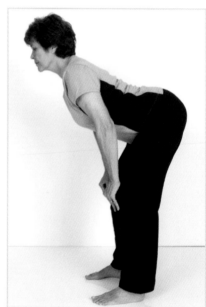

STANDING FORWARD BEND (*UTTANASANA*) WITH BLOCK, ALTERNATING LEGS

I find this alternating leg ... *satisfying and almost painless. In the following steps, you will experience immediate imp...*

YIN TIP: *Th*... *something to support your body weight as you bend forward fr*... *yoga block (available in most sporting goods stores). Th*... *latform and helps you hold your poses longer. (See* ... *assist you with your poses.) If you are not very* ... *weight supported by your hands on the block.*

- ... *gs.* ... *the ham-* ... *ront of your* ... *breaths. Now* ... *the block directly in* ... *body weight into your right* ... *leg* ... *ed; it is soft and comfortable.*

- Now str... ...t leg, keeping your left foot on the floor. As you hold... ...reathe, slowly lift your left shoulder up toward your left ear. Enjoy the stretch; feel it start and end. Then walk your hands to the center and repeat on the opposite side, placing the block in front of your left foot.

- Finally, return hands to center. Observe that your hamstrings, hips, and lower back have released, and your hands are closer to the floor.

- The three Rs can be applied from this position. To Resist, gently press your hands into the support. Hold for one or two breaths. Release, Relax, and Restretch. Finally, after you've straightened one leg at a time, try both legs at the same time. It will intensify the move. Lift your sitting bones. Your head hangs like an apple on a tree. Come up slowly, as your head is filled with more blood circulation than usual; you may feel dizzy if you come up too fast. Halfway up, use your feet, thighs, and legs to return to standing.

Knees to Chest (*Apanasana*)

Benefits: *Soothing for the back. Increases abdominal circulation.*

- Lying down on your back, bring both knees in toward your chest. Clasp your hands below your knees.

- Exhaling, open your knees slightly and press them outward over your ribs (not over the center of your chest). Inhale, then release, still holding on to your shins. Repeat, going back and forth, three to six times, aiming your knees toward your armpits.

Yin Tip: *Guiding your knee more to the side of the body creates space in ligaments and tendons, thus avoiding the sensation of hip compression. If you have knee problems, hold the backs of your thighs.*

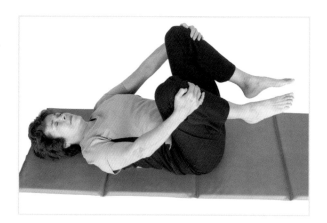

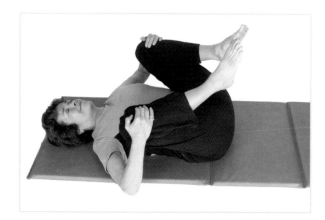

Seaweed Legs

BENEFITS: *Warms up legs and hips for standing poses.*

- Begin in Knees to Chest pose. To stabilize and support your lower back, place your wrists beneath your sacrum (the base of your spine) to "make a nest." Straighten your legs, and shake them out for 10 seconds. This shaking actually helps muscle fibers to soften and releases tension.

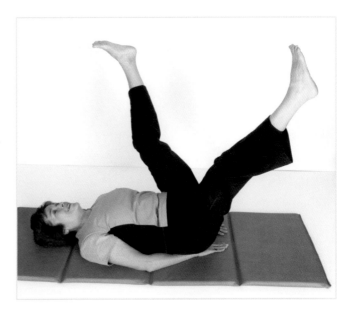

- Now pretend your legs are like two giant strands of seaweed moving gracefully in all directions with the warm current of the sea. Be creative: two legs moving separately, bending and extending in all different directions for three to six breaths. Enjoy!

- Then pause. Bend your knees, and place your feet on the mat. Close your eyes, allowing time for your witness to observe how your legs feel. Connect with the pleasure and fun of doing Seaweed Legs.

KNEE TO CHEST WITH THREE RS (*VAKRANASANA*)

This warmup is an old friend because it is such an effective, beneficial warmup for all postures. However, Knee to Chest is a bit misnamed because the knee is aimed not so much toward the center chest but toward your armpit and the side of your ribs.

BENEFITS: *Good warmup for hips. Soothes the lower back and increases circulation for internal organs and leg muscles.*

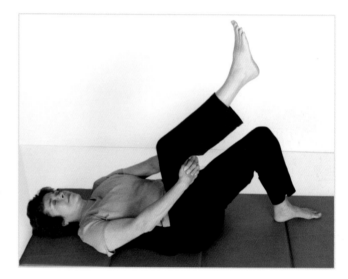

- Lie down on your mat on your back, with feet to the floor and knees bent. Bend your right knee into your chest with hands clasped behind your thigh or over your knee. Now incorporate some warming up movement. Inhaling, slowly push your thigh away from your chest. Your elbows will straighten. Then, exhaling, slowly press your thigh to your chest, aiming for your right armpit. Go back and forth in rhythm with your breathing, six to eight times.

- Now add on the three Rs. Keep the right knee bent and the lower leg passive. Resist . . . press your thighbone into your hands while your hands push back to form a little wall of resistance. Hold the resistance with a steady pressure for three to six breaths. Relax, breathe in . . . feel your body relaxing. Exhaling, Restretch. Press the thigh closer toward the side of your body . . . relax your shoulders and jaw . . . hold for two or three breaths. Then repeat on the opposite leg.

WALL CALF STRETCH

BENEFITS: *A tight calf muscle (gastrocnemius) can limit hip movement. This is my yin warmup version of the popular runner's stretch. Take it in steps and you'll feel immediate painless results.*

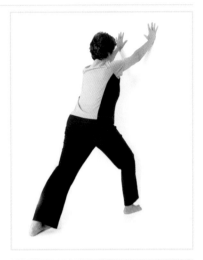

- Place your right big toe close to a wall, bending the right knee. Then take a long stride back with your other leg. Look down, and make sure both feet form a straight line forward and your right knee is over the ankle. Place your hands on the wall for support. Gently root your left heel to the floor. Hold this preliminary stretch for 10 quiet breaths.

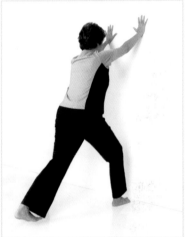

- The three Rs are achieved by bending your left knee, pressing the ball of your left foot into the floor, with the heel slightly lifted. Resist . . . lean your body weight into your hands on the wall . . . feel the resistance in your arms, upper body, and left leg as the ball of your left foot presses into floor . . . hold gentle resistance for 10 breaths. Relax . . . breathe in . . . exhaling, Restretch.

- For the final stretch, Relax, breathe in, and Restretch. Exhaling, press your left heel to floor . . . roll your weight from the little toe toward the big toe . . . pull your kneecap up . . . hold for 10 to 15 easy breaths. Try keeping your shoulders down and heels relaxed. You may find that after the three Rs, your elbows and upper body will move closer to the wall. Repeat the steps on the opposite leg.

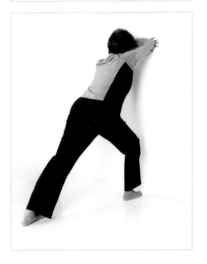

YIN TIP: *The calf muscle and the Achilles tendon together carry the weight of the body. No wonder they are both strong and tight! I recommend holding the final step a longer time to achieve a pain-free, highly effective stretch.*

Barn Door: Piriformus Stretch (Supta Ardha Padmasana)

A tight piriformus muscle (it's the one you'll feel stretching when you do this pose) is the normal condition of most beginning yoga students at midlife. It contributes to mild stiffness and the inability to bend forward with ease from the "hinge" of your hip. But here's a big CAUTION: Hip pain can be caused by a very tight piriformus pressing the sciatic nerve against the pelvic bone. Stretching while you are in pain due to sciatica is possibly not helpful. Please seek direction and advice from your health practitioner. Otherwise, this level 1 piriformus stretch is fabulous for opening your stiff hips. Go slowly, and listen to your body. My yoga friend Crista Ripin calls this the cowabunga muscle. You know when that muscle is being stretched and can yell, "Cowabunga, I found it!"

- Lie on your mat faceup, with knees bent and feet to floor. Place your right ankle on your left thigh; now look at your bent leg. Be sure your ankle is sufficiently supported by your thigh. Imagine your knee is a barn door that needs to be opened. Place your right hand on your right knee and press open the knee as if opening a door, three to six times. Hold open for a few breaths.

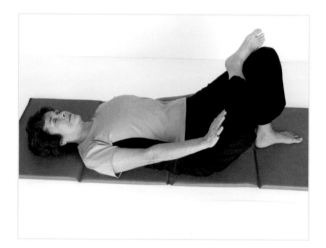

- Now, reach your right hand through your legs and hold the back of your left thigh. If you cannot reach this far, use a belt around your left thigh and gently pull it toward you. The right hip muscle that you feel stretching is the piriformus. Practice the three Rs, keeping your back and hips to the floor. Press your right ankle into your left thigh, your hands pulling your thigh to your chest, forming a gentle wall of Resistance. Feel the hip muscle being activated as you Resist, holding for a count of five. Pause. Breathe in.

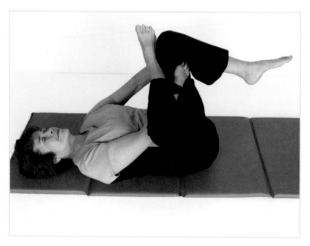

Relax. Feel your hip and legs relaxing. Exhaling, Restretch. Slowly pull your left leg closer to your chest. Aiming your left knee toward your left shoulder, keep your back and hips on the mat. Hold for three or four breaths.

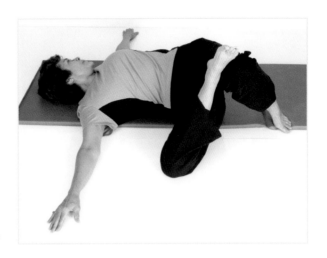

YIN TIP: *For flexibility and proportional reasons, your shoulders and head might come off the mat while you try to hold this pose. Place a pillow beneath your head or use a belt around your thigh. It will help you to relax and hold the pose.*

- Side/Side Variation: With your left foot on the floor, your right leg is in Barn Door. Your arms are in T position. Slowly let your right leg fall to the right, and look over your left shoulder. Now return to center and repeat on the opposite side. Force nothing. Hold for two or three breaths. Release, and come out of the pose.

HUG A TREE

BENEFITS: *This is an excellent warmup for all standing poses. A comfortable yet powerful hamstring stretch, this stretch is different than simply bending forward. After a few times, my students experience significantly improved flexibility in their hamstrings.*

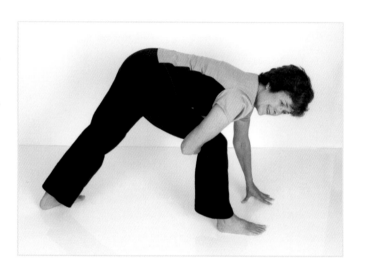

● Begin in Sacred Mountain Pose, but with your feet wide apart. Turn your left foot in and your right foot out. Bend your right knee about 90 degrees. Turn your torso toward the right and fold forward over your thigh. Your chest will touch the thigh. Place your left hand on the floor, close to your right foot for balance. Wrap your right arm around your right thigh and "hug" your thigh.

● This is a great place to do the three Rs. Start gentle Resistance by trying to lift your chest away from your thigh, yet keeping tight contact between them. Your head lifts, and your back stays long. Hold for three breaths. Relax . . . breathe in. Exhale . . . go deeper into the pose, Restretching the leg without losing chest/ thigh contact. Repeat on the opposite leg.

YIN TIP: *As you progress, begin to straighten the practice (forward) leg without sacrificing the body/thigh close position.*

DOWNWARD-FACING DOG WITH A CHAIR

BENEFITS: *Combines the benefits of partial inversion and bending forward, and helps remove a lifetime of stiffness from the upper body. If you have trouble kneeling or getting down and back up from the floor, you can enjoy this pose very early on into your practice. A weight-bearing pose, it sends a stimulating message to the arm bones to retain calcium, thus helping to prevent osteoporosis.*

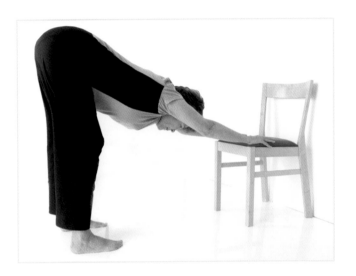

- Put a sturdy chair against a wall. Place your hands shoulder-width apart on the front edge of the seat, then take big step back. You are a full arm's length from the chair, with your heels slightly behind your hips and feet hip-width apart. Your body forms a little V. Press your hands firmly into the chair seat, evenly distributing your weight between your hands. Lift your heels off the floor . . . your bottom is high. Exhaling, press the chair into the wall, lengthening your spinal column. Focus on your comfortable, calm breathing.

- Now do Dog Wag by moving your hips and ribs from side to side. Firmly press your heels, one at a time, into the floor, and spread your toes. Smile; enjoy the stretch. Come out of the posture, and step forward toward the chair. Slowly stand up, then sit down in the chair. Let your arms hang, close your eyes, and take a restful 30-second vacation.

STANDING FORWARD BENDS (*UTTANASANA*)

BENEFITS: *These bends lengthen the entire back body and make space between the vertebrae of your upper neck. I like these poses, as you will soon see, because they are very versatile. Gravity helps free the cervical spine and allows the neck muscles to relax, improving overall circulation and having a calming effect on the body and mind.*

CAUTION: *Be very careful of all forward bends if you have disc problems. If you have any questions, check with your doctor or health professional.*

- Start in Sacred Mountain Pose (page 54), with your feet slightly apart, your shoulders down, and your hands in Namaste.

- Inhaling, raise your arms forward, then up overhead, arching your back slightly.

- As you exhale, sweep your arms out to the sides and bend forward from your hips. When you feel the pull on the back of your legs, soften your knees.

- Let your arms hang and touch earth ("earth" could be a block or chair in front of you). Ease your knees just a little more to relax your lower back.

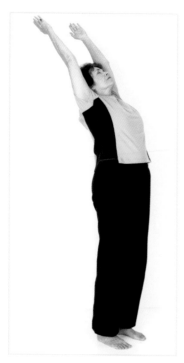

- As you inhale, roll up slowly, and then raise your arms overhead. Repeat the steps three more times. Then stay in the folded position. It feels relaxing to fold your elbows and allow the weight of your arms and torso to gently stretch your body toward the floor. No bouncing! No

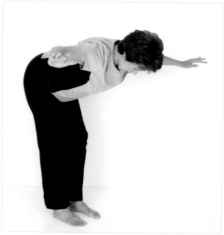
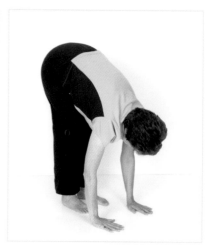

strain! To come up, place your hands on your legs and walk up. Be sure you continue to breathe. Stand tall.

YIN TIP: *If leg and back tightness makes this position really uncomfortable, practice with your elbows or hands on a chair seat or other support.*

● Variation: In the first step, keep your bottom against a wall, then step both feet forward about 12 to 16 inches, according to your flexibility and height, with your feet hip-width apart. Exhale, and fold forward as you go through the steps.

SPIDY ON THE MAT

● Start in Table Pose (page 143), on your hands and knees with your shoulders aligned above your hands and your back straight. Very slowly, sit back on your heels, giving your ankles a chance to stretch out. Then, folding over your thighs, extend your arms way out in front of you as far as possible. Open your knees so you can breathe comfortably. Breathe in and exhale slowly, enjoyably, letting your trunk sink close to floor. Hold for two to four breaths.

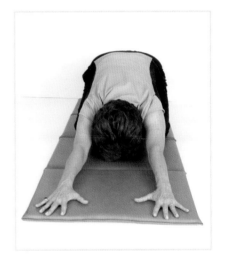

● Slide your right hand beneath your right shoulder. Focus your attention on your left straight arm. Now walk your left hand like a little spider, to the right. Your left upper arm will come close to your left ear. Do not move your head. Pause here, breathing comfortably. Feel the wonderful stretch from your left hip to your fingertips. Hold for 30 seconds. Enjoy the stretch. Walk your fingers center, bring your right hand back up, and repeat the stretch on the other side.

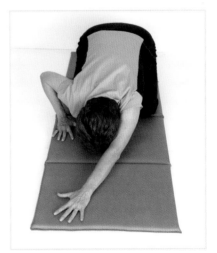

LITTLE MERMAID SERIES

This pose is named after Denmark's Little Mermaid statue, inspired by the Hans Christian Andersen tale.

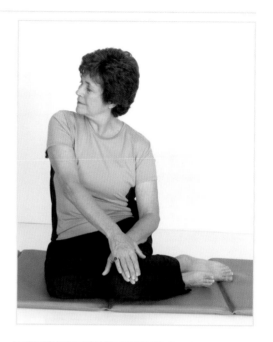

- Sit on your mat with your knees bent in a double V off to your left side. Rest your left ankle on the arch of the right foot. Secure your left hand to your thigh with your right hand, and look wistfully out to sea over your right shoulder.

- Inhaling, raise your right arm. Exhaling, extend the arm into the space to the left. Hold the stretch for two or three breaths.

CAUTION: *Remind yourself to stay in a comfortable range of motion for your hip and knee.*

YIN TIP: *This delicious stretch fits perfectly into preparing for the Pigeon and Standing Dancer poses.*

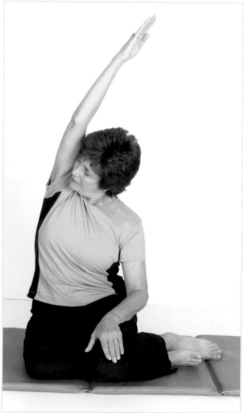

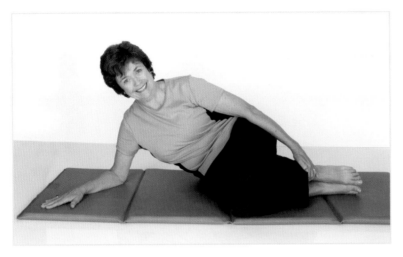

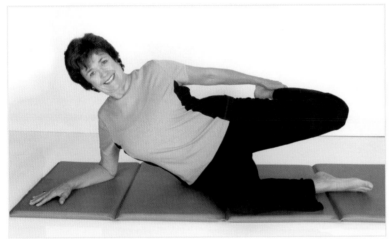

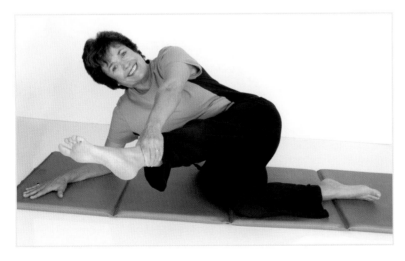

● Place your right forearm to the floor. Your knees are still bent, and your hip "hinges" are bent at about a 45-degree angle, stacked directly over one another. Reach with your left hand to grab your left ankle.

● Slowly exhaling, pull your left leg comfortably back. Take a moment to look at your left knee. It should stay parallel to floor. Gently pull your left shoulder down and back. Hold for two or three breaths. Enjoy this stretch.

● Inhaling, draw your left leg out in front of you, changing the position of your hand on your ankle. Exhale and swing your extended leg out in front of you then across your chest for two or three breaths. Repeat three or four more times, then repeat on opposite side.

ROLLING PIN SERIES

BENEFITS: *The following playful rolling moves will enhance flexibility, release restrictions of soft tissue, and increase all-over body circulation. Use your own body weight to give connective tissue a massage. I often find the Rolling Pin Series extremely nurturing. It makes me smile and brings a laugh to the class.*

- Begin in Knees to Chest pose (page 62), but bend both your knees, wrapping your arms around your legs or the backs of your thighs. This is called *Apanasana*, or Wind Reliever pose, because it does just that. If you hold in intestinal gas, this posture will release it. Please don't be embarrassed if this happens to you in class. It's a common occurrence—I'm just relieved it has never happened to me on TV! If needed, use a belt on the back of your thighs. This helps to loosen neck and shoulder tension. Exhaling, allow the weight of your arms to draw your thighs toward your chest and the weight of your torso to melt the lower back to the mat. The back of your head stays on the mat, shoulders down. Close your eyes and imagine with the next inhale your entire spine lengthening from skull to tailbone. This is a comforting, peaceful pose. Stay in it for a few more breaths.

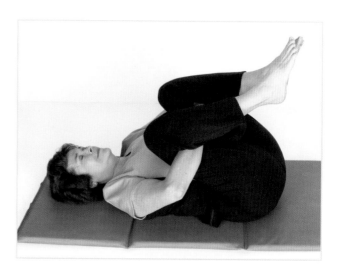

- Now become a Little Boat by introducing a gentle rocking movement, side to side, while staying in Wind Reliever. Comfortably and mindfully rock right elbow to left elbow, side to side. Don't forget to go onto your shoulders and upper back.

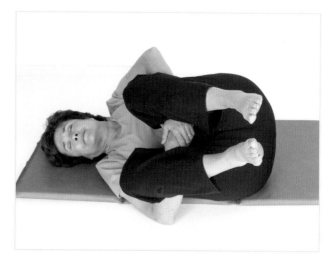

- Variations:

Play a little. Let your head follow the direction of your knees and body, then turn your head in the opposite direction.

Try wrapping your arms around your upper body and give yourself a hug, continuing to roll from side to side. This move helps release deep shoulder tension.

Try extending your arms over your head while rolling side to side. Place your feet on the floor to stabilize your body, and roll slowly from side to side.

- Hip Rolls: Sit on your mat, knees bent, feet flat to your mat. Place your hands on the floor behind you and lean back, supporting your weight with your arms, lifting your feet a few inches off the mat. Your body weight rolls past your tailbone and onto the flat part of your lower back called the sacrum. Now roll slowly from side to side over your seat muscles and up your outer hip. Feet are off the floor as you continue gently rolling side to side, *not* on the tailbone. Try playfully extending one leg out, then the other, as you roll. Do this for about a minute, or as long as feels comfortable.

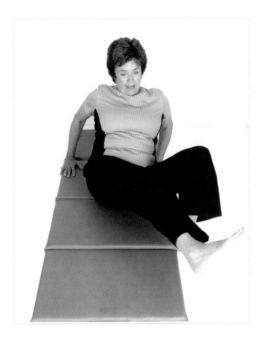

- Facedown Rolling Pin: Roll over so that you are facedown on the mat, your hands on the mat beneath your shoulders for support. Roll side to side on your abdomen. Then use your arms to slightly lift your upper body and roll side to side on your thighs.

- Now try the full Rolling Pin. Begin lying on your back with your legs straight. Then extend both arms up and over your head, upper arms close to ears. Slowly roll completely over onto your abdomen. You probably will roll off your mat onto the floor, which is fine. Then roll back to the center of your mat and, like a rolling pin, roll completely over to the other side. If you feel adventurous, do a few more rolls over and over, each side. Have fun. Rest quietly for 1 minute.

FILL THE CUP

BENEFITS: *Gives a gentle squeeze to the liver. Warms up side waist, thigh, and leg muscles.*

- Stand tall in Tadasana, Sacred Mountain Pose. Focus your attention on your right hand. Turn your palm up, fingers forming a cup. Fill this cup with feeling and awareness. Inhaling, raise the cup of feeling up over your head.

- Lean to the left side as far as you comfortably can. Slide your left hand behind your back to your right hip. Your upper-body weight is completely supported on the left hip.

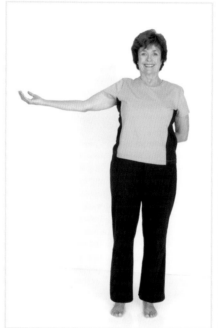 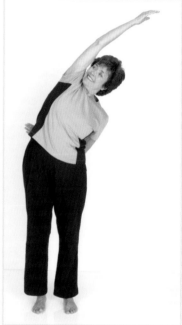

- Extend the right arm out a little more into the space to the left and pour out the cup of feeling. In one smooth motion, turn your chest toward your left, rolling your shoulders, and look down at the floor, sweeping your right hand to the floor in front of your toes, easy on the knees.

- Inhaling, slowly raise the cup of feeling. Come up to standing. Repeat two or three times, moving slowly and gracefully. Then repeat on the opposite side.

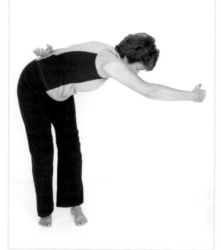 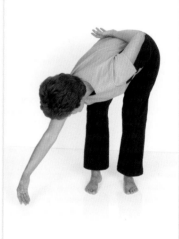

VICTORY GODDESS (*DEVIJAI UTKATASANA*)

This delightful Victory pose resembles the dancing mythic gods and goddesses from the Hindu tradition. It is both a warmup and a posture full of joy and wisdom, reminding us not to take ourselves too seriously—a reminder that practice is meant to be wise and fun! Ancient yoga masters must have been aware of the stress and tension we humans collect and carry in the neck and face. Scrunching our eyes and mouth, opening our eyes wide, and stretching out the tongue really help facial and jaw muscles to relax and release physical and mental tensions.

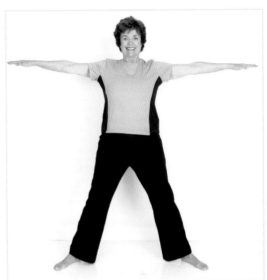

- Begin standing in Sacred Mountain Pose, feet close together but not touching, breathing comfortably, eyes soft, hands in Namaste (see page 174). Inhale and step your left foot to the left, about 3 feet away. Turn both feet out slightly. Pause, exhaling. Inhaling, sweep your arms out from your sides, making them parallel to floor, palms facing down. Your body forms Five-Pointed Star.

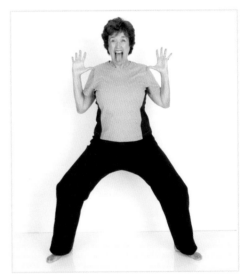

- Exhaling, scrunch your eyes and purse your lips. Bend your knees, going into a comfortable squat. If possible, your calves and thighs should form a right angle, but only go down as far as is comfortable for you. Bend both elbows, placing your thumbs on your shoulders. Inhaling, lift your chest and stretch the palms of your hands. Now, exhale forcefully, and go a little deeper into the squat. Open your eyes wide . . . lift the brows . . . stretch out your tongue. Hold for two breaths. Release, and repeat these steps three times.

- On the third time, hold the posture when your body forms Five-Pointed Star. Close your eyes and mouth. Focus your inner attention on your pelvic bowl. Drop into the flames of your own power and wisdom. Feel the fire leaping and crackling within you. Stay for a breath or two. Smile. It feels good and empowering as you fan the flames of wisdom. Release the posture, and return to Sacred Mountain Pose.

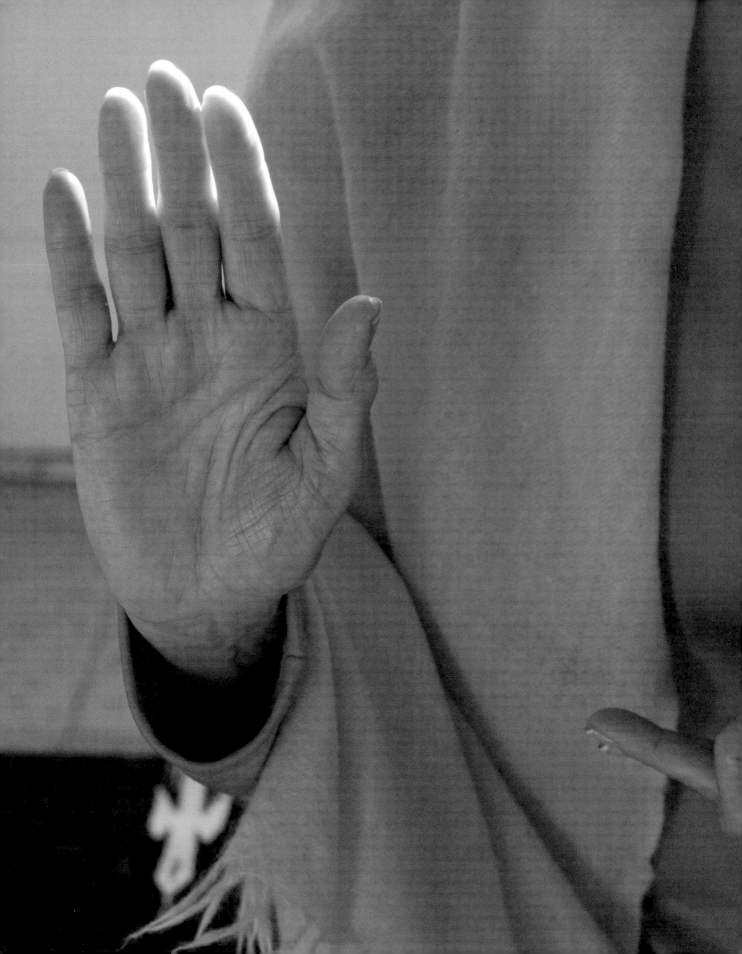

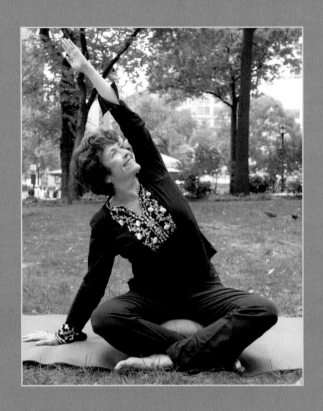

PART FOUR

PRANA-MAYA-
KOSHA

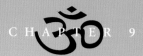

CHAPTER 9

YOUR ENERGY BODY

The physical body, discussed in Part Three, is simple to understand. Nobody has trouble relating to it. Now we move into the other koshas, which are a little further removed from our everyday thinking. The second "body" is the *prana-maya-kosha*. *Prana* is associated with our breathing. This is your "breath body," sometimes called the "energy body."

While it is closely associated with the physical function of breathing, this kosha is not considered to be primarily a "physical" part of ourselves. It's a sort of human energy field made up of our mental, emotional, psychological, and spiritual currents.

Traditions of the East and West share the belief that every human being on the planet has this secondary, nonphysical energy body. Ancient Egyptians called it "ka." Yogis called it "prana." Plato called it "the form of things." For centuries, artists have painted this energy body as a radiant, golden halo or nimbus around the heads of sages and saints. Development of this, and all the koshas, leads to a deeper cooperation with your body's capacity for healing and knowing.

It is possible to see it with your own eyes.

Modern Kirlean photography can capture on a special type of film this aura that radiates from all matter. But beyond technology, many people can see auras, especially in highly energetic or charismatic people. I experienced this when I was honored to be a faculty member at a conference where President and Mrs. Carter were also teaching. All of us watched the door in expectation, as Mr. Carter was a little late for his class. Finally, the door flew open. Within a millisecond, all I could see was a huge, gold, brilliant flash of light spreading out in all directions. Then Jimmy Carter, with his endearing smile, walked into the classroom.

This energy, or prana, is likened to fuel that feeds and circulates through the physical body and mind, in the same way that our breath does. When it ceases to function, the physical body—

heart, lungs, brain—stops working. Cells disintegrate. We strongly identify with our material body, yet without support of the nonphysical prana sheath, we cannot survive. Pranayama, our breathing practice, enhances the circulation of prana to all levels of the koshas.

Have you noticed that some people give you energy? You feel happier, even healthier, just being in their company. I'm sure you've also had the opposite experience: after a certain person has left the room, you feel tired, exhausted, and drained, as if run over by a Mack truck. It could be following an encounter with a friend, a client, or total stranger. It could happen over the phone or face-to-face.

A powerful example of the latter happened to me many years ago. Highly respected author and yoga teacher Bo Lozoff asked me to accompany him to Ohio's maximum-security Lucasville Prison. Bo has been teaching yoga to men and women in the penal system throughout the United States for more than 3 decades. For me, it was my first and only time to be locked into a prison. I had no idea what to expect.

Our class consisted of 25 men. Bo spoke eloquently about the philosophy of yoga. I was to follow with some stretches and relaxation techniques. About halfway through his talk, I realized I was feeling weird. The best way to describe it is

by recalling the demise of the Wicked Witch of the West in the *Wizard of Oz*: "I'm melting," she cried pitifully after being splashed with water. I felt as if 25 invisible straws were siphoning my energy and I was slowly melting down.

The experience was frightening. My energy pump was definitely on empty, and I had no idea how to fill 'er up! Desperation helped me to dig deep for tools. As Bo finished his talk, I closed my eyes, slowed down my breathing, and with each breath visualized golden light surrounding and filling the empty inner spaces. To my relief, with each spoken word, the energy began to move through me once again.

Pranic energy can be transmitted in many ways—through a genuine smile, a voice full of compassion and kindness, the touch of a hand upon your shoulder. It can also be affected by the negative, angry, or suspicious energy of others. We can influence the flow of our pranic energy by focusing on specific, positive thoughts (as I was able to do in the prison) and by intentionally changing our breathing patterns. Yoga devotees use a series of breathing techniques called pranayama to exercise, refuel, and replenish vitality to *prana-maya-kosha*. The next two chapters will help you become familiar with pranayama and give you specific instructions for trying it yourself.

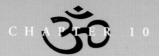

CHAPTER 10

INTRODUCING PRANAYAMA

Before you begin this chapter on pranayama, I want you to know that these pages are a mere drop in the bucket of breathing. My recommended books on breathing are listed in Appendix B. The authors of those books are respected yoga masters who share with us every possible nuance of this most sacred subject, the breath. Prana is a concept that means energy or life force. Although not specifically the breath, prana is usually associated with breathing since, without our breath, we don't have life.

Entire yoga classes are devoted to exercising the energy or breath body. The exercises, such as diaphragmatic breathing, complete breath, and crocodile breathing, are called pranayama. The meaning of pranayama can be confusing. It is often referred to as "controlling one's breathing." But, if pranayama is to be understood, it is as two words: *prana* and *ayama*—to lengthen or to stretch. In pranayama, we purposefully extend or shorten our breathing patterns with the intention of affecting the flow of our prana.

Yoga masters teach us that breath is not prana, nor is prana air. If that were so, we'd be pumping air into a dead body to revive it. You cannot see, touch, or directly manipulate prana. We use different, interesting breathing rhythms like a lever to work indirectly on the prana, thus keeping energy moving well throughout our daily lives.

Prana is closely linked to breath and life, because we enter this world on an inhale and will depart this world on an exhale. Illness could be looked at as the improper flow of prana, and the absence of prana is death. Prana exists in all living things. I personally feel that all of nature—trees, mountains, river, even rocks—is breathing.

There are many assumptions and stereotypes associated with yoga breathing, so let's go through some of the "is nots." The purpose of pranayama is not to hold one's breath for as long as possible, nor is it to awaken a serpent of energy coiled at the base of your spine. It is not to produce levitation nor to come out alive after being buried for days.

So what *is* yoga breathing? Learning to observe your own breathing patterns and to be able to switch from one that produces tension to one that produces relaxation is a great beginning. There are numerous specific techniques, and I'm going to teach you a few of them. But first, let's discuss some breathing basics.

BREATHING TRIVIA

Let us begin with the humble nose, an impressive asset in your arsenal of power tools for health. There is something a little comical about the ol' proboscis. It doesn't enjoy the dignity or respect of the eyes or mouth, and many folks are dissatisfied with the size and shape of their nose.

The nose performs 30 vital tasks, including these: We breathe 18,000 to 20,000 times a day, at the rate of 12 to 18 times per minute. The nose filters air, moisturizes, provides a tunnel for oxygen, creates mucus, and serves as the drainage passage for the sinuses. People who live in hot, humid climates tend to have wide, open nostrils because moist air needs less processing. People in cold and very dry climates seem to have longer, narrower noses, perhaps to warm the air or filter the dust.

You have an outer nose and an inner nose. The internal nose is connected to the brain and nervous system. The inside of the nose is bumpy, lumpy, and cleverly designed to direct and move air toward the inside of your head before it travels into the lungs.

Every 2 hours or so, one nostril becomes more dominant than the other, thus alternating and reversing the airflow. Western scientists call this natural biological alternating flow "infradian rhythm." You can try it right now. Close one nostril with your thumb and slowly inhale through the opposite nostril. Switch sides and repeat. Try it one more time. Observe which side feels slightly more open. Check back again in 2 hours and I'll bet you that the open side has changed.

Modern science continues to explore the link between breath and emotions. Researchers confirm intuitive wisdom of the past that by consciously changing your breathing patterns, you can shift emotional states. Studies show that the length, depth, and rate of the breath have a powerful effect on the brain. Of course, yoga breathing began thousands of years ago, long before we had scientific data to substantiate its effectiveness.

By lengthening your exhalation, you can:

▶ Clear your mind
▶ Quiet your inner dialogue (or inner talking)
▶ Better control fear, anger, anxiety, and pain
▶ Ease into sleep
▶ Increase vitality and sexual pleasure
▶ Improve concentration

- Ease pain and stress of childbirth
- Calm your own nervousness and the nervous energy of people around you

I think I'd better explain that last one. The next time a friend or family member is upset or nervous, notice his or her breathing; it's probably erratic, shallow, and high in the chest. Now, purposefully slow your own breathing down as you listen to the person's story. It might take a few minutes, but often this little technique helps you to stay cool and will influence the other person to calm down. I used this years ago when my children were upset. Today it is a practice I use often with my grandchildren. It has also come in handy on airplanes when my seatmate is a nervous flyer.

A good place to begin is to focus on the exhalation. You can try this right now, where you sit, by practicing a Bramari, or Humming, Breath. Two or 3 minutes of this lengthening of your exhalation can provide a real time-out from tension.

Bramari Breath

Begin by closing your eyes. Tune in to your friend, the witness. For 1 minute, observe your "everyday breathing." This is breathing master Richard Rosen's term for how we normally breathe out there in life. Choppy, uneven, shallow one moment, smooth and long another moment—that's normal, everyday breathing. Listen to its sound, but do nothing and change

nothing. Just allow the witness to observe, watch, and be curious.

Place your hand, palm down, over your navel or belly area. Place the other hand on top of it. Just observe, feeling the belly expand and flatten for the next 10 breaths.

On your next exhale, begin to hummm. This hummm is not a chant or a song. It is more of a sustained tone. I love using sound because it establishes a focal point and gives a little resistance to help control your exhalation.

Begin the hummm . . . slow, even, and comfortable. Inhale quietly . . . now do another long hummm. Feel your closed lips vibrate. Your tongue floats in your mouth, and your jaw muscles are relaxed. Unclench your teeth. Inhale . . . now another long exhale: hummm. No struggle. This time, gently pull in the navel area during the last few seconds of the exhale. Allow the next quiet wave of the inhale to start itself. Effortlessly, the wave flows in, then again the long exhale. Repeat this exercise 10 to 20 times, finding a comfortable rhythm for you. For variation, aim the sound of "nnnn" into the back of your skull to refresh your brain. Practice with "sss" or "eee" sounds. Have fun! Practice in the shower, at stoplights, or immediately after a stressful moment has passed.

THE ANATOMY OF A YAWN

Everyone on the planet yawns. Can you picture that? The whole human race, soul to soul, uses the humble yawn to ventilate the body. Even the animal kingdom yawns. (I secretly wonder if butterflies and snakes yawn, but I've found no concrete evidence either way.) Just thinking about the subject makes me want to yawn right now. Keep reading—you'll feel it too!

Many years ago I discovered the spontaneous yawn to be one of the most simple, pleasant, and effortless yoga breathing practices.

Listening to your own body, notice that the clue begins with an inner low-pressure swirl somewhere in the back of your throat and head. Soon, the swirl nudges you to open your mouth and stretch from the inside out: the jaw, tongue, nostrils, larynx (vocal cords), and bronchial tubes.

Without you thinking about it, the eyes squeeze closed and tear ducts release their soothing liquid. The shoulders lift, and we raise both arms up and rock side to side. Intercostal muscles, located between the ribs, lengthen and the diaphragm lowers, allowing space for a deeper breath to rush in. The heartbeat quickens, and blood flow to the brain increases. Sometimes even the ears gently unblock.

All of this takes less than 6 seconds! Notice how you feel afterward. Tingly energy travels through the body; yawning sends a blast of energy to the brain.

The yawning reflex is mysteriously connected to health. People who are seriously ill or suffer from severe psychiatric disorders do not feel the need to yawn. When my students yawn in class, I know it's not boredom or impoliteness. It is the body's signal to "*feed me*."

Now stop reading and take a time-out. (I don't recommend yawning in public because we all know how contagious it is.) Witness your conscious, enjoyable yawn. Open your mouth wide, squeeze your eyes shut, lift your arms above your head, straighten one arm and then the other, inhale deeply, chest open, and then let out a good, loud exhaling sound, like a lion. Nobody can hear you! Go for it! Exaggerate this wonderfully simple, mystical yawn. At the end, pause; close your eyes to let a long breath roll in and out of your body. Bring as much feeling as you can into both the right and left sides of your body.

Some people have a difficult time stopping the yawning reflex. Here is an option. Let the swirling effect start, then consciously exhale slowly, slowly out. Picture your breath going down into and through the heels, soles, and toes of your feet. As a lightning rod channels excess energy into the ground, you can channel the excess yawn downward to be absorbed into the earth through your feet.

The yawn is an example of a type of breath that's a little different from everyday breathing. Like yoga breathing, it serves a purpose. Are you ready to try some pranayama? The next chapter will show you how. I have experienced everything I'm about to share with you about breathing. I've been fascinated by it and found that it truly enhances and brightens my health and emotional balance in midlife. I can't wait to share it with you!

CHAPTER 11

TIME TO BREATHE

In this chapter, I'm going to show you several specific yoga breathing techniques: Three-Part Breathing, eyes of your heart breathing, alternate nostril breathing, and Kapalabhati. I'll finish with a particular breathing pose. Before you learn about the various techniques, I want you to read a few pointers about breathing in general below.

NINE TIPS FOR HEALTHY BREATHING

1. During your day, take a breather . . . it's the pause that refreshes. Many yoga breathing techniques can be done sitting in a chair wherever you happen to be.
2. Until a receptacle is emptied, it cannot be filled. Until we breathe out fully, it is impossible to breathe in correctly.
3. Do all breathing (unless you're asked to do otherwise) through your nose, not your mouth.
4. Keep your jaw, tongue, and facial muscles soft, and shoulders down from ears.
5. Listen to the silence of your breathing. Hear its flow . . . silent . . . smooth, silky breath.
6. If you can hear yourself inhaling, you are trying too hard. Don't try to inflate yourself like a tire or balloon.
7. Exhaling should be easy, effortless, silent, and deep.
8. Be aware that leather belts and underwire bras can hinder respiration.
9. Relax. . . . Relaxation is the open door to breathing.

THE PRACTICE OF BREATHING

THREE-PART BREATHING (DEERGHA SWASAM)

BENEFITS: *Whenever you feel tired, depressed, or discouraged, do Three-Part Breathing. Utilizing your full lung capacity takes in seven times the amount of oxygen that normal shallow breathing does. It keeps lung tissue elastic, steps up your metabolism, and reduces tension and anxiety.*

PART ONE

- Lie on your back with your knees bent and feet on your mat (or bed), hip-width apart. Place a pillow beneath your head to relieve neck tension. Tilt your chin downward slightly.
- Place your right hand on your belly, with your thumb resting on the navel (this area is called your belly area). Close your eyes; it will help you become aware of your belly as it lifts and lowers . . . rises . . . and falls.
- Begin the inhalation by expanding the belly. Feel the lower lungs fill. As you exhale, contract the belly muscles in. Inhale . . . expand the belly . . . exhale . . . contract the belly. Continue until you feel comfortable and familiar with the practice of part one. Notice how this simple practice of belly breathing makes you feel calmer and more relaxed.

PART TWO

- Keep your right hand on your belly and left hand on the side of your ribs. Now exhale completely through your nose, all the way down to the "basement" of your breath.
- Inhale, expanding the belly. Continue to slowly inhale, expanding the lower rib cage.
- Then exhale, allowing the breath to flow out of the mid-rib area and middle lungs . . . pulling in the muscles behind your belly area.
- Inhale . . . expand the belly and mid-rib cage. Then, exhaling, contract your ribs and, last, your abdomen. Continue parts one and two of Three-Part Breathing until you feel comfortable.
- End part two with an exhalation and return to your normal everyday breathing. Enjoy the quietude.

PART THREE

- Exhale . . . now inhale . . . expand the belly . . . expand mid-ribs . . . continue to inhale to the "ceiling," filling your upper chest. Feel the collarbone rise slightly.
- Exhaling quietly and slowly, release the air from the upper chest, lower chest, and belly.
- Repeat Three-Part Breathing three to five times.

You may not use your chest muscles and lungs to their full expansion. If you feel dizzy—stop. If you begin to strain, get tired, or short of breath—stop. Return to everyday breathing and rest. After resting, continue Three-Part Breathing a few more times. This will help you build your stamina. Once you get comfortable with Three-Part Breathing in the prone position, experiment with sitting up tall. Observe the differences between prone and sitting erect. Adjust to seated Three-Part Breathing, since you are upright much of the day. Breathing in this way will soon be automatic if you practice it on a daily basis.

EYES OF YOUR HEART BREATHING

"Where are the eyes of my heart?" you might be asking. Place your fingertips on your chest below

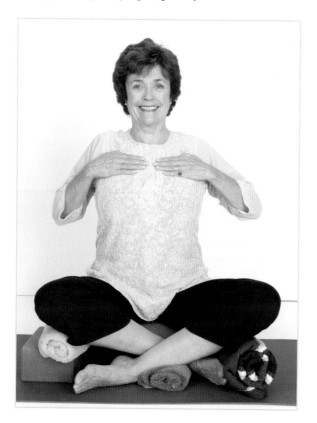

your collarbone. Pretend you have two great eyes that open on the inhale and stay open on the exhale. Feel it happening. You'll read cues to lift up your heart or open the eyes of your heart in many warmups and what I call Desert Island postures. Now, let's breathe, still resting your fingers on the eyes of your heart.

- Using Three-Part Breathing, inhaling, imagine your heart eyes opening wide, looking up to the ceiling. Smile.
- Exhaling, keep them open in wonder and delight.
- Inhaling, open the eyes further. Exhaling, breathe slowly, quietly, as air flows out. Keep your heart eyes open as long as possible. Continue for three to five more breaths.
- Breathing with wide-open heart eyes prevents the old habit of the chest collapsing on the exhale.

ALTERNATE NOSTRIL BREATHING

Yoga masters have known for hundreds of years that we don't breathe evenly through both nostrils. My experience has been that the blocking up of one nostril for more than 4 hours could be a signal of a head cold coming on—or that my mind could use a break from thinking or needs some emotional balance.

Alternate nostril breathing (ANB) is an exceptionally effective technique for calming and relaxing both mind and body.

- Sit comfortably, spine tall, in a chair or on a pillow on your mat.
- Place your left hand in your lap. With your right hand, make a gentle fist. Release your thumb, little finger, and ring finger. This is a classical hand position called *Vishnu Mudra*.
- Place your right hand so that your thumb closes the right nostril. The little and ring fingers will close the left nostril. Index and middle fingers are tucked against the ball of your thumb.
- Close off the right nostril with your thumb. Inhale slowly and comfortably full through the left nostril.
- Close off the left nostril with your fingers, and exhale through the right nostril.
- Inhale through the right. Close off the right nostril with your thumb and exhale through the left.
- Continue this pattern. Exhale, inhale, switch nostrils. Exhale, inhale, switch.
- Repeat ANB practice 10 to 15 times.

Once that feels comfortable, try inhaling while mentally counting to 5 on the inhale and exhaling silently while counting to 5. No strain. Work up to practicing ANB for 1 minute. Finish your last exhale through your left nostril.

At the end of a minute, place your hands in your lap. Close your eyes, and dive inward. The witness is there quietly watching, observing. Reconnect with stillness, the peaceful place within.

If you feel uncomfortable, stop ANB and resume normal breathing. As lung capacity improves, make your inhale and exhale longer. Never force the breath. Gradually increase ANB to 3 minutes a day.

KAPALABHATI

Kapalabhati (pronounced kah-pah-la-bhah-tee) means "shining the skull." This technique is high on my favorite breathing list. Kapalabhati makes the sound of a broom sweeping back and forth, so I like to visualize a broom sweeping my front brain, nasal area, and lungs clean and clear of all debris. Practice in the morning, not before bedtime. If you get light-headed, stop and slowly do Three-Part Breathing.

In the first step, you will use the open-mouth vowel sounds of A-E-I-O-U. Sounds help the brain to understand, focus, and experience this wonderful technique. The kid in you might find it fun, too. Spend time in step one. Get comfortable with the mechanics. Then move on to the second step, with your lips closed.

- This energizing technique emphasizes the exhale through the nose with short, staccato-like breaths. But first try it with the A-E-I-O-U sounds and an open mouth. Relax your abdomen on the inhale through the nose . . . on each vowel sound (the exhale), pull your navel in . . . A-E-I-O-U. Repeat. Keep watching the emphasis, navel in, the sound, and exhale. The inhale just happens.

- Sit tall. With a tissue close at hand, establish Three-Part Breathing for 1 minute. Lips are closed, teeth unclenched. Nearing the end of your exhale . . . contract muscles behind your navel . . . observe that more air is pressed out . . . relax . . . notice air flows in without any effort on your part.
- Now, take that information and exhale again. Quickly pull the abdominal wall back with one powerful, sudden action, as though you are trying to expel debris from your nose. Relax your facial muscles and passively allow the air to flow into your lungs. This is one Kapalabhati breath cycle. Repeat this seven to 10 times.
- By emphasizing your forceful exhale, the inhale relaxes. Notice you can take in a longer inhale. Keep the repetitions rhythmic. Begin with 10 reps, done in sets of three, with time to breathe normally between sets.
- I love practicing Kapalabhati with certain postures and before my meditation practice. It truly helps quiet the restless mind.

CAUTION: *Your stomach must be empty. If you have high blood pressure, heart disease, or experience dizziness, best not to include this in your pranayama practice. Remember, when in doubt—don't!*

CROCODILE BREATH

If you have been a chest breather (and most of us are during the day) all your life, Crocodile Breath will automatically shift you into breathing diaphragmatically. Diaphragm breathing enables you to feel well and clear, maintain emotional balance, and reduce fatigue and stress. This technique combines three-part and belly breathing. You can translate Crocodile breathing into moments seated at your desk. Take a breathing break—while sitting in your car, standing at the bus stop, watching the evening news, even soaking in the bathtub.

- Be comfortable. Lying on your belly, place a pillow beneath your chest and under your ankles. This pose can be done facedown on your mat, in your bed, before sleep, or to help you get back to sleep.
- With each inhale, you are doing a little pushing-up of 15 pounds of body weight, thus toning the flabby diaphragm muscle easily and painlessly.
- Cross your arms in front of you. Place one hand over the other to form a pillow. Rest your forehead on your hand-pillow. Nose points toward floor. Neck is long.
- Begin by closing your eyes, and for 1 minute watch your breathing from this upside-down position.
- Inhaling, observe the belly pressing against the earth (that's the pushup).
- Exhaling, observe the belly pulling away from the earth.
- Inhaling . . . belly swells . . . ribs expand; feel the earth's energy filling your body and mind.
- Exhaling . . . let the earth absorb any worries, concerns, thoughts, and emotions that keep

you from feeling peaceful and at ease. . . .

- Continue for a few more minutes. You might even fall asleep in this pose.

A GIFT FROM YOUR BREATH BODY

To close this chapter, watch and observe your breathing pattern when something upsetting or stressful occurs in your life. It can be a very simple event. The car alongside you, without warning, cuts in front and you jam on the brakes. Without thinking, you inhale sharply, you clutch the wheel, and your gut contracts.

Stop reading this page for a moment. Imagine you are tooling down the highway, the car cuts you off, and you put on the brakes. What happens to your breathing? Imitate your breath. A sharp, quick, eyes-open, high-in-the-chest in-breath. Yes! Consider that quick little in-breath as a *gift*—a pop of energy that allows you to clearheadedly handle the incident. That high pop of energy served you well—it assisted you through the stressful moment. But if it stays there, high in the chest, for years, it becomes a problem. With yin focus, bring the breath down low into your pelvis. Lower your shoulders. Inhale, open your mouth, and exhale three nice, long, mellow, let-go sighs, inhaling in between them. Smile and feel your whole body relax.

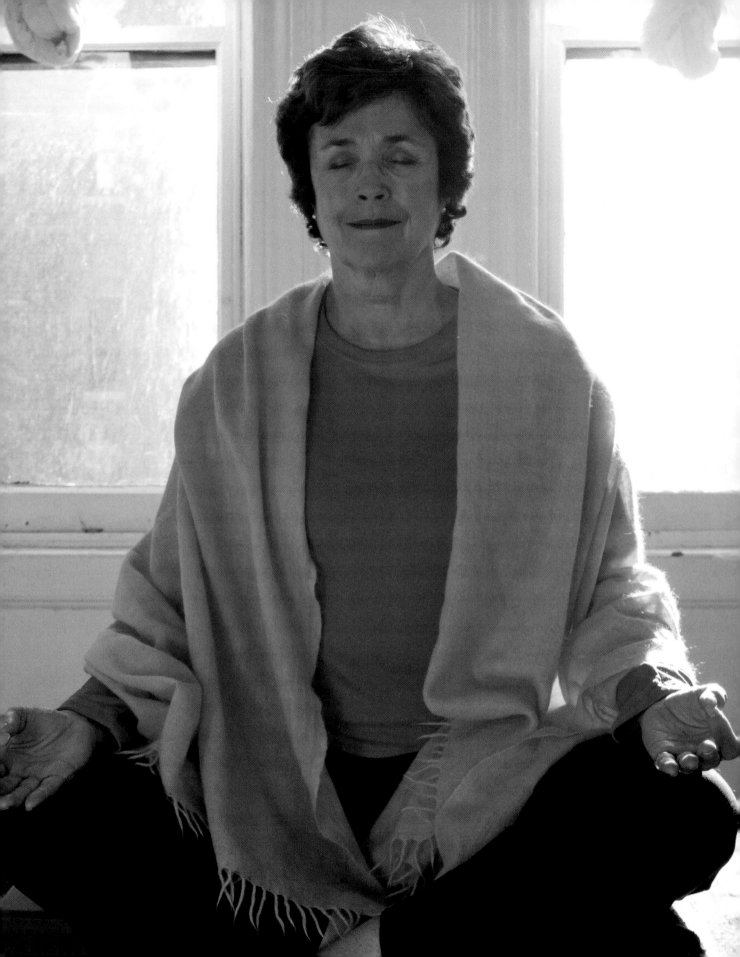

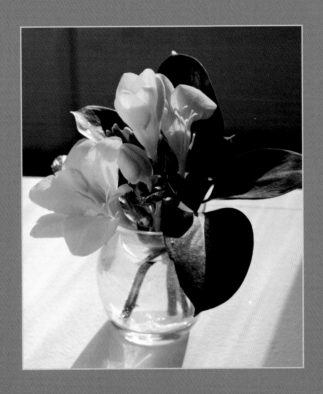

PART FIVE

MANO-MAYA-KOSHA

CHAPTER 12

YOUR MENTAL/ EMOTIONAL BODY

"ANY GOOD YOGI WILL TELL YOU, SUFFERING, OLD AGE
AND DEATH DON'T AUTOMATICALLY VANISH WHEN YOU
CAN ARCH BACK AND TOUCH YOUR HEAD TO THE SOLES
OF YOUR FEET."

—*Anne Cushman, in the* Shambhala Sun

The first two koshas we discussed were all about the physical body and the breath body. But you know you're so much more than that. You're also a person full of thoughts and feelings and emotions. The third of the five koshas is the mental/emotional body. In this body we store everything we have learned, felt, and perceived. All sensual perceptions—tastes, smells, favorite songs—are stored in this body called the *mano-maya-kosha*, meaning "body made of thought process."

As our physical body carries physical scarring, our mano-maya-kosha carries the scars of past wounds, stressful thoughts, memories, hurts, and pains. A physical scar might remain where you cut your finger 5 years ago, but emotional wounds from 40 years ago form the mental scar tissue of today. As we age, our mano-maya-kosha becomes increasingly burdened with all the stress and injuries of our past. At this time of life, it's more important than ever to take care of our mental/emotional body.

One of the benefits of yoga is its power to soothe the body, quiet the mind, and balance the emotions. Breathing and relaxation techniques are enormously helpful in keeping your mental/emotional body healthy. Strengthening your witness and detachment helps to keep you in balance.

The mental body feeds on the energy of obsessive, stressful thinking and the sense impressions we offer it. If we keep supplying our third sheath a continual stream of violent news; stressful, agitated thinking; and conflicted relationships, the mano-maya-kosha begins to crave increasingly aggressive forms of this insidious energy. One of the best things we can do for our mental/emotional body is to be careful what we feed it.

YOGA AND OUR THIRD KOSHA

Sure, there are moments of a blissful buzzing after doing the deep back bend of Camel Pose (page 151). There is a profound, mellow calm at the end of long relaxation. The world can look and feel very different upon leaving a weeklong yoga retreat. Even the roadside debris and billboards glow with light and love.

But sooner or later we hit the wall of hard stuff. We find our ability to touch our palms to the floor absolutely useless in the face of emotional habits like selfishness, fear, and irritability that are so deeply ingrained in the mano-maya-kosha. It is common in yoga class to uncover old injuries, whether to our heart or our hamstrings. I often ask myself, what is the point of experiencing the peace found in relaxation and meditation, if I can't maintain it for 5 minutes after I'm finished? I may feel great in yoga class, but why can't I heal the rifts with my own family or friends?

From the moment we step on the yoga mat, we come face-to-face with ourselves as we actually are. It's our biggest challenge and our greatest joy.

People ask about the difference between feelings and emotions: Are they the same? I don't think of them in the same way, even though we often use the words interchangeably. I think of emotion as experiencing a particular state of consciousness, such as fear, joy, or sorrow. Emotions fly out in all directions. Feelings are more linear and calm. They do not do battle with things and emotions. In fact, feelings can help control emotions. In midlife yoga, the goal is to move through life with less battling of emotions and more into a pure state of feeling.

I was in the midday of my life before I truly admitted I was tired of carrying ancient, emotional pain like a dead, stinking donkey everywhere I went. Midlife is the time to say, "Enough of pain!"

But when it comes to emotional pain, the only way out is through. You have to feel it to heal it. This is a tall order for most of us humanoids. Recent studies show that emotional pain registers on the "Richter scale" of our brain as real physical pain. During my time in psychotherapy in my thirties, I likened talking about and reconnecting with old emotional pain as being operated on without anesthesia.

The good news is that your body was born to know what to do with pain through crying, weeping, breathing, and moving. When we were babies it came naturally, but as we grew up we learned to suppress this natural process as a sign of weakness.

The gift of midlife is being mature enough to understand that there are kindly, safe, and nurturing ways to heal your own emotional pain. Allowing yourself to feel fully "what is" is a great beginning. As you identify and express emotions naturally, you open the door to releasing the pain.

I've found this to be true again and again, as I've dealt with my own personal demons. Finding and making space for those scrunched-up emotions, fears, and anxieties is probably the most difficult and challenging inner work I've ever done. It's taken maturity and time to feel the freedom that comes from facing, not re-burying, painful memories and emotions. This place where we store all the stuff we'd rather not feel seems remote and safe—but it actually affects our everyday lives, robbing us of peace and the freedom to enjoy life. Spiritual teacher Eckhart Tolle calls this place the "pain body."

THE IMPACT OF THE PAIN BODY

Standing in my kitchen a few years ago, two very dear married friends were intensely discussing ancient grievances within their relationship. I sat at the table, trying not to take sides and hoping for the right words to help the situation. My friend Mary shared her deep hurt and fiery frustration. Her whole body, face and arm movements, tone of voice, and words expressed her anger. Her husband, Ben, sounded restrained and calm; his limp body language looked cucumber-cool.

There came a moment when I thought I might say something insightful. Knowing that it can be healing to at least be in touch with what you are feeling, I naively said to Ben, "You might not look it, but I think you are very, *very* angry." He turned toward me, saying calmly, "I . . . am . . . *not* angry." And as the words came out of his mouth, little black arrows, like dark, sharp porcupine quills, flew out of his body, aimed in my direction, hitting my belly like a pincushion.

At the time, I didn't understand this experience, but it was real. I could physically feel his anger hitting me. I received some insight from Dr. Norman Shealey, founder of the American Holistic Medical Association. "There are sappers and zappers," he explained. A zapper is someone who is indiscriminately angry, like my friend Ben. They let it fly, so to speak. You can feel it in your body—particularly your chest and belly—when you've been zapped. It's not personal, but it still hurts.

Sappers, like my experience of the men in prison in chapter 9, are the folks who cannot get enough. There is a great hole that will never fill. You can give and give, but it is still nowhere near enough. Usually these people are quite depressed. Their mano-maya-kosha feels empty.

My experience with Ben was a vivid example to me of how our mano-maya-kosha, even though we can't see it and it seems abstract, affects every bit of our lives. Everything we store there comes out somehow. It even affects those around us. Whatever we have in our mental/emotional body may seem hidden, but in reality it can have a profound impact on everyday life.

Some people may not feel it's important to tap into their thoughts and emotions, particularly if it involves experiencing negative feelings or delving into the past. If that describes you, you may want to skim over this section and come back to it later when you're ready to give it a try. But if you're like me, you may be tired of carry-ing your emotional baggage with you wherever you go. This journey of exploration into yoga will help you lighten your load.

While I am talking about the yoga approach to healing the mental/emotional body, I want to acknowledge that these yoga-related practices should weave together with other work you may be doing to find peace in your inner life and in your relationships. Personally, I could not have made it this far without the help of traditional psychotherapy. There are times when we need to use a variety of methods to uncover and release old pains so we can move into the future unfettered. If you're suffering from any type of depression, anxiety, anger, conflicted relationships, or other peace-robbing difficulty, I encourage you to seek the help you need in the form of a counselor, psychotherapist, or spiritual advisor. You will find that the yoga approach in this section can simply enhance your process of healing.

TAKING THE FIRST STEP TOWARD HEALING

I've found that healing my pain body involves, first, recognizing its existence, and acknowledging the emotions that reside there. Personally, one of my greatest challenges is fear. I need to take my time to safely look at a fear, experience its energy, and realize in my heart of hearts that I am not going to succumb to this experience. I picture my fears looking like gorillas. I have 5-pound gorillas, but there are 500-pound gorillas, too. Today nobody is asking me to tussle with my 500-pound gorilla! However, one of my 25-pound gorillas is my fear of heights. Lying belly down at the edge of 3,000-foot cliffs in Montana is terrifying. What if the cliff should crumble? (After all, it's only been there for a few thousand years!) What if I fling myself over the edge? (Sorry folks, I have a vivid imagination.) Over the years, I've found that using techniques such as relaxation, breathing, and visualization helps me tame this fear.

As you sit reading this book, are you aware of any negative emotions dogging you? Stress that won't go away? A fear or anxiety that seems to weigh you down? Sometimes we wrestle with lifelong gorillas. Other times it's just a normal, day-to-day worry that sits on our shoulders.

Either way, I've found it helpful to begin dealing with these joy-stealers by going through a process of acknowledging them and symbolically letting them go. Following is an exercise that helps me do this.

You can do this brief routine whenever you're feeling overwhelmed by the stuff in your pain body. Does it magically make the pain disappear? No, of course not. But it can help you get in touch with exactly what that pain might be, and give you the tools to begin the process of releasing it.

NAMING AND RELEASING YOUR PAIN

- Sit up tall in a chair and close your eyes. Reconnect with your witness self. Remember, there is no judgment in the witness and nothing so awful that the witness cannot see it. Scan your body. Your feet are connected and supported by the earth mother.
- Focus on your breathing. Soften the jaw muscle. Take a slow long breath in . . . long, slow, quiet breath out. Repeat three or four more times . . . knowing that holding your breath or shallow breathing prevents you from fully feeling. Long, slow breaths help you to feel and dissolve the pain.
- Take a moment to name your pain. Describe it as fully as possible in writing or out loud. Don't sensor yourself. See the memory with its accompanying pain clearly. Just tell the truth to yourself about what it is because what is not acknowledged cannot be healed. Place the emotion into your hands. Give it color and shape. Call your pain "the pain" instead of "my pain." This will make it easier to let go.
- Now slowly lift the pain up with your two hands. Yes, actually raise both hands upward, travel across your chest, your throat, your forehead, and now lift the pain above your head. Hold it there.
- Imagine there is a glorious yellow flame above your head. Ignite the pain with the flame. See it flare up brilliantly. Let the emotional dross burn for a minute or so.
- Lower your hands, leaving the ash residue to continue to burn above your head.
- Sit for a few moments. Dive inward. Observe the spacious, quiet sweetness that has been created. Enjoy it for a minute longer. Close by thanking yourself for being willing to take your time and attention to your pain, plus bringing more lightness into your life, your family, and the world.

Releasing the pain is not a onetime event. It is a process done again, and again . . . and yet again.

CHAPTER 13

CONNECTING WITH YOUR MENTAL/EMOTIONAL BODY

"TO MEET EVERYTHING AND EVERYONE THROUGH
STILLNESS INSTEAD OF MENTAL NOISE IS THE GREATEST
GIFT YOU CAN OFFER THE UNIVERSE."

—*Eckhart Tolle*

The year was 1966 and Swami Chidananda was speaking in New York City at the Sivananda Yoga Center on 13th Street. It had been an extraordinary week for me, a housewife and mom from Norwalk, Connecticut. To spend so much time with a saintlike man from India was a gift I did not quite understand at the time.

This day in New York, we were all sitting in a circle around the swami, listening to some uplifting yoga discourse charged with his special brand of wisdom, humor, and love. I'm sure I had reached my saturation point of spiritual discussion, so I sat in the circle, a blissful lump, and looked around at the people in the room. My eyes paused and I peacefully looked at a woman sitting across the circle from me. From a quiet, silent place inside my head, I heard myself say, "I'm prettier than she is." It took me a few shocked seconds to realize and register the content of this murky thought. Here I was, sitting at the feet of my teacher, in a state of high bliss. How could I possibly have such low thoughts? But there they were, traveling across my forehead like ticker tape on Wall Street.

It took me a while, but my experience that day taught me a profound lesson: I am *not* my thinking. What a huge relief! I do not have to be at the beck and call of every thought that floats through my head. Just because I'd had that stray, distasteful thought didn't mean I was defined by it. I didn't even have to pay it any attention.

This can be a breakthrough in how many of us treat our mano-maya-kosha—the mental/emotional part of ourselves. Rather than be a slave to it, we can choose how much power to give it. We can choose whether or not to develop a thought. With practice, you'll soon catch yourself smiling at the antics of what the yogis call "monkey mind"—where your mind seems to have a mind of its own! But you can learn that you don't have to take the contents of your mind so seriously.

In fact, there are a number of techniques we can use for staying connected with our mental/emotional body. Visualization is one of them.

I literally stumbled, or I should say fell, into visualization. Picture this: I was a tall, lanky 14-year-old, wearing red ski pants on the icy slopes of Vermont, tangled in my skis, weeping in frustration. All day long, my family waited patiently for me to untangle myself. Finally they'd had enough. Off they skied, leaving me to get down the mountain on my own. In the car on the drive home, my father said, "Lilias, if you don't change your attitude, no one will want to ski with you ever again."

Pouting in teenage silence, I remember thinking, "No one will ski with me? I'll show them!" Motivated by anger and pride, I began to picture myself skiing. Each night before sleep, I'd close my eyes and daydream. On the movie screen behind my forehead, I saw myself, happy and smiling, carving turns, hearing the skis whoosh against the snow, seeing the blue sky, smelling the crisp air. This daydream went on throughout spring, summer, and fall.

The following winter, my family watched with apprehension as I stood on the crest of the beginner slope and pushed off. I skied down perfectly, smooth turns and all. "What happened to you?" my dad asked later. I had no idea how to answer him then, but today I do. The months of visualization had made all the difference.

Visualization, also known as imaging, is a valuable tool for many reasons, but especially for creating and maintaining good health. Reams of scientific articles attest to the value of visualization techniques. It is used for self-improvement (enhancing athletic performance, quitting smoking), therapy (conquering insomnia, relieving depression), healing (of immune system disorders, cancer, and injuries), and pain control.

Visualization can be a special kind of language between body, mind, and soul—a language full of sound, sensations, images, smells, colors, and taste. Because imagery involves activating particular circuitry in the brain, it is easy for some and challenging for others. If the "muscle" of visualization has not been used for a while, it can become weaker with age. But you absolutely can develop it at any age with regular and devoted practice.

I recommend using visualization to help with any physical, mental, or emotional challenge you're facing. It is amazing how much we can control our behaviors and responses through this tool. People with a little bit of experience in visualization can be quite effective at quieting their minds with even a tiny visualization, as the following story illustrates.

There are layers of stillness. I first made this discovery teaching evening yoga classes. Night classes are filled with hardworking men and women who sit in front of a computer or talk to people on the phone all day. Tired and eager to begin class, they dive for their yoga mats. The room becomes quiet.

It was in that quiet pause before the class began that I noticed a buzz in the room. The room was completely quiet, yet I could still hear a sound. It dawned on me that the staticlike buzz came not from an air conditioner or radio; it was from the energy of thinking thoughts! The outer room was quiet, but the inner rooms of heads and brains continued to talk like transmitters, causing this buzzing static.

As soon as I gave a brief visualization of letting the day go, the mental noise stopped. The minds went into neutral gear and relaxed with ease, spontaneously dropping into a deeper layer of stillness.

It is this deeper layer, this place of stillness within us, that we strive to reach as often as possible, to keep our mano-maya-kosha as healthy and peaceful as possible.

CONNECTING WITH YOUR EMOTIONAL BODY

GENERAL VISUALIZATION

- Create a pleasant, quiet environment. Take the phone off the hook. Close the doors. Keep warm. Turn on soothing music or environmental sounds.
- Sit or lie down in a comfortable position. Maybe place a pillow beneath your knees, head, or curve of your neck.
- Close your eyes softly . . . connect with your witness self . . . feel where your eyelids touch . . . turn your inner gaze upward toward the movie screen of your mind. Pause at the ellipses . . . involve your senses.
- Daydream . . . of a lemon . . . its skin texture, color . . . its smell . . . cut open . . . see the pulp of the lemon . . . now take a bite . . . (long pause) . . . let that image dissolve . . . .
- Daydream of an apple . . . its color . . . rub it on the sleeve of your shirt . . . feel and hear the rubbing . . . now look at the apple shine . . . lift it to your nose, smell the apple . . . now take a big bite . . . hear the crunch . . . feel the juice dripping from the corners of your mouth . . .
- Let the image dissolve. Daydream of the ocean . . . smooth ocean . . . now choppy ocean . . . waves moving in all directions . . .
- Dissolve the image into stillness . . . and now hear the wind in the trees . . . rustling the leaves as it travels through . . . .

Visual or auditory, do what comes naturally. There is no right way. More suggestions:

- Approach each practice session positively.
- It is very important to practice before a major

problem develops that could be helped by visualization. Practicing visualization and relaxation is like putting money in the bank. It's there when you need it!

- Approach each practice session positively. Expect to have a good time. You're a very okay person, someone lovable, right now in this present moment. If negative thoughts come ("this won't work"), visualize them written on a blackboard and then erase them. Watch the words fade.

- Practice often. This is a skill that sharpens with use. Be patient.

- Consider obtaining audiotapes on relaxation, which are excellent tools for learning the fundamental skills. You'll find some of my recommendations listed in the back of the book.

- Expect the unexpected. This is a right-brained, nonrational activity.

CAT AND MOUSE EXERCISE

This is a variation of an exercise from author and philosopher Eckhart Tolle. It's a great way to strengthen your consciousness and stay in touch with your mano-maya-kosha.

Close your eyes. Sit tall. Take a moment to watch your breathing, changing nothing. Gaze upward, to the space above your nose. Daydream. Imagine you are a cat sitting outside a mouse hole, waiting for a mouse to appear (Tom and Jerry come to mind). Feel your stillness,

your quiet, active focus. Then silently say to yourself, "I wonder what my next thought will be?" And wait . . . silent as the cat, for the next thought to come out of the hole.

GET OFF YOUR TRAIN OF THOUGHT

Here is a way to step lightly off your train of thinking.

- Close your eyes. Focus your attention on breathing through your nose. Simply watch your effortless breathing in and out. Note that it feels cool when you breathe in, warm as you breathe out. Simply observe, witness. Cool in, warm out.

- Focus your attention above your nose, in line with your eyebrows. Daydream of a beautiful mountain stream flowing by. Hear the sound . . . see the little rivulets of water flowing over stones. Wait until the next thought wants your attention. Then turn the thought into a brown, moss-covered log. Let the log float by. Choose not to develop the thought; just let it float downstream.

- Once again, see the stream, clear, running free, easy . . . wait for the next log or thought to come to your awareness. Choose again not to develop that thought. The thought floats by . . . only the stream remains.

- Practice for 1 minute. Extend, as you can, to 2 or 3 minutes.

The Waterfall Visualization

Water is a powerful symbol of purification. Sit tall with eyes closed. Daydream . . . recall a picture of a beautiful waterfall. Let the picture come to you . . . see yourself standing under the waterfall. Now feel the power of the water on your skull, spilling across your shoulders and down your legs. Hear the sound of the waterfall in your ears, washing your whole system, through your whole body. Visualize the water washing away negative thoughts, impurities of the day; wash out your feet into the stream below. Envision what it means to "let the day go."

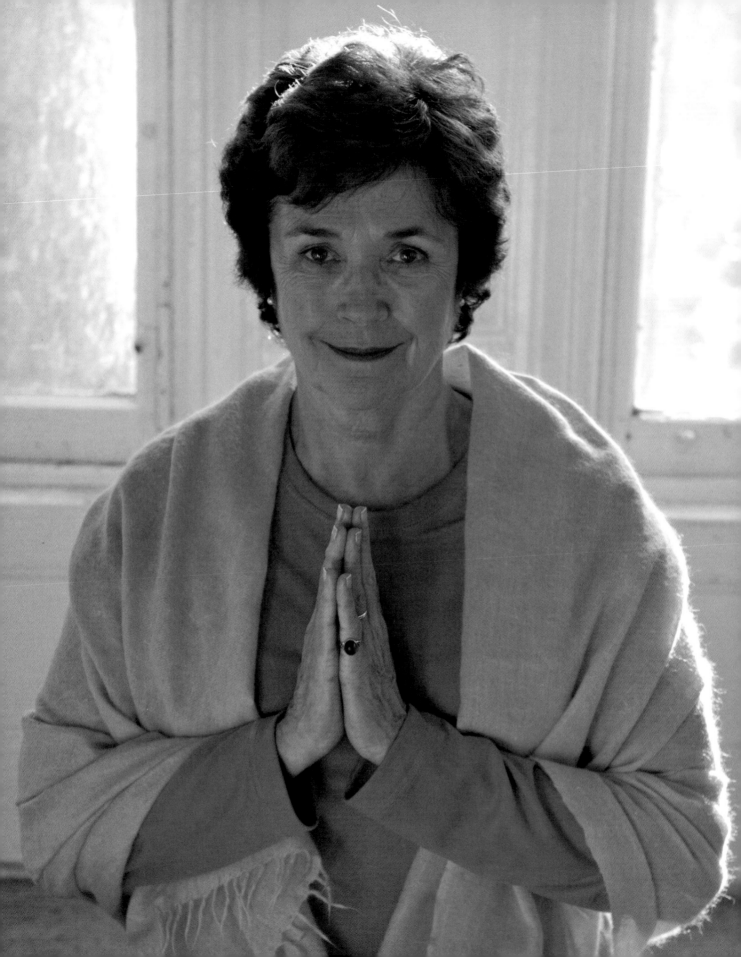

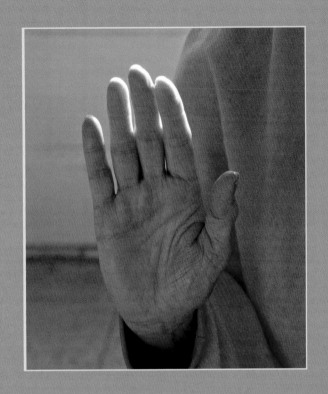

PART SIX

VIJNANA-MAYA-
KOSHA

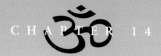

CHAPTER 14

YOUR WISDOM BODY

Your fourth sheath—even subtler than the mental/emotional body—is called *vijnana-maya-kosha*. This is your body of higher wisdom, judgment, and discernment. It is an interesting word to pronounce. Give it a try . . . . Make the "j" sound like a "g" as in "fig": "vig . . . nana." There you go. Vijnana.

Developing this kosha means tapping into your deep inner reservoir of knowledge and intuition. This is where your willpower lies. This is where you get your strength of character. The more you nourish this layer of yourself, the more you'll be able to trust your own judgment and decision making. You have spent a lifetime building your wisdom body, but less time intentionally cultivating it and purposefully accessing it. At midlife you will probably find it tremendously rewarding to expand your self-awareness by taking steps to nurture your fourth kosha.

I find it easier to understand this sheath when I look at the areas of my life in which I notice that my vijnana body is clearly underdeveloped. Can you think of stressful moments when you've had a hard time making up your mind, thinking for yourself, or being creative? Times when you've had little willpower or been the victim of your own poor judgment? You may notice this in other people, too. Some people show weakness in their fourth sheath in their lack of personal ethics or conscience, or by difficulty discerning right from wrong.

We often associate "wisdom" with "thinking." Of course, it's the nature of our minds to think! But wisdom goes deeper than our thoughts. A giant step toward understanding the wisdom body is realizing, "I am not my thinking." We need to find ways to get behind our thinking and penetrate our deeper wisdom.

One way we develop our fourth kosha is with the help of the witness. Take your witness by the hand and reflect on your lack of willpower or indecisive moments. (Remember, no judgment—just observe.) What decisions give you difficulty? For me, sometimes it's as simple as my difficulty saying no to a jelly doughnut. I've got a real weakness for them. My witness helps me recognize my weakness for jelly doughnuts and for saying no!

Strengthening your wisdom body is empowering. It's like finding a wise inner warrior, and together you meet life's challenges. The following exercise will give you a fuller sense of your wisdom body:

First, read this paragraph . . . sense the part of your awareness that consciously decided to participate in this exercise and is commanding you to sit quietly and finish it. Close your eyes, focus your attention in the center of your head, and for 1 minute sense that part of your awareness . . .

Continue reading . . . sense that part of you that recognizes the value of self-awareness . . . close your eyes. For 1 minute, sense that part of you that recognizes the value of self-awareness.

Reading on . . . sense the part that compels you to rise early in the morning to do your yoga and meditation practice . . . close your eyes. Sense for 1 minute that which compels you to get up for practice.

Reading on . . . now sense that part in you that confronts laziness in wanting to stay in that warm bed rather than practice. Close your eyes . . . confronting the laziness. The part of you that is doing the confronting . . . this is your vijnana-maya-kosha.

with a group of friends or family members. Everyone stands up and turns to the next person. Next, look each other directly in the eyes and firmly say, "Yes! I can!" to each other.

Now turn to someone else . . . be aware of the energy exchanged between you. Look into the second person's eyes and say, "Yes! I can!" Think about your willpower that needs strengthening. "Yes, I can unblock my creativity!" Say it to someone else . . . really mean it. "Yes, I can make decisions!" Experience the power of *Yes!* in your body—pump your fist, stamp your foot, create a ruckus. Find one more person, look into his or her eyes, and say with conviction, "Yes! I can!"

This exercise can also be done solo. Just turn to the mirror and look at your image and say, "Yes! I can! Yes! I will!" When you look at yourself in the mirror, your eyes unite with your brain, tapping into the rich connections with your emotions and your physical body. The affirmation "Yes!" helps us to go deeper and connect with vijnana-maya-kosha.

Each "Yes!" helps me find inspiration and dig deep to grasp the energy to give one more yoga class. Yes, I can say no to a jelly doughnut or do my yoga practice even when I don't feel like it. Yes, I can!

AN EXERCISE TO CONNECT WITH YOUR WISDOM BODY

"Yes" is a great power word. We can use *Yes!* as a way to strengthen the wisdom body. This exercise can be fun and noisy and empowering to do

USING MEDITATION TO CONNECT WITH THE WISDOM BODY

Another very powerful and effective way to connect with your wisdom body is through meditation.

"What is meditation?" a student asked me as we took an autumn walk. "Is it brainwashing?" I must admit the question stopped me in my tracks. Brainwashing techniques do not have a great reputation here in the Midwest.

Then I began to think about it. Yes! Brainwashing could be one way of looking at meditation. Each morning I try to "wash" my brain free of worry, agitation, fear, and other stressful emotions. Meditation leaves my brain clean, fresh, calm, and clearer.

When you are not burdened with surface worries and anxieties, you are better able to come closer to your deepest wisdom. That is the goal of meditation. But anyone who tells you that meditation will stop your thinking doesn't understand the process. Meditation will teach you how to skillfully *manage* your thinking. It is a huge relief to know that not every thought needs to be developed.

Research shows that meditation is good for your physical and emotional health. Several studies reported in *The New England Journal of Medicine* beginning in 1976 to 1977, found that relaxation techniques—meditation among them—are very effective stress-management therapies. Since then, doctors, hospitals, and clinics worldwide have increasingly recommended and taught relaxation and meditation to patients, especially those with high blood pressure and heart disease.

Some people are skeptical of meditation, but they do recognize the benefits of a relaxation exercise or a power nap. Actually, there are similarities among all of these therapies. They all slow down your blood pressure, heart rate, and breathing. But when meditators are hooked up to an electroencephalograph (EEG) machine, brain waves are slowed, and right and left brain patterns are balanced. This does not occur in sleep or other relaxation techniques.

At midlife, you have a large reservoir of wisdom available to you, should you decide to tap it. I hope that in the following pages you find practical tips and encouragement to support your first steps toward beginning meditation. Some of the brilliant masters of meditation and breathing are listed in the back of this book. Read something that uplifts the spirit and feeds your soul.

Before you begin to meditate, there are some steps you can take to prepare. You'll want to carve out time and space for meditation, and you'll want to prepare your body and mind. I've jotted down some thoughts and expanded a few ideas that have helped me in my own path to meditation.

PREPARING YOUR TIME AND SPACE FOR MEDITATION

1. CREATE A SACRED SPACE. Choose a space in your home that inspires you: a place that, each time you walk by it, calls to you and reminds you of the deep peace within you. It could be a

corner of a room or even a walk-in closet, where you put a meditation pillow, a blanket, and your yoga mat. I have a special table with a candle, flowers, and inspiring pictures of family, spiritual teachers, dear friends, and beloved animals that have passed on. This is a place to put anything uplifting that encourages you to remember the joy, peace, and sacred stillness within.

2. CHOOSE YOUR MEDITATION SEAT. Traditionally, meditation is done on the floor, but you may be comfortable in a chair (feet on a pillow if needed), in bed, or on the floor with a pillow. Create a seat where you can sit erect. You need to be comfortable, free from distractions and pain.

3. CARVE OUT TIME. Choose a convenient time for you and your lifestyle. Many people meditate when they first wake up. Others like to meditate before sleeping or at a certain time of day. It's best to find a time that will work consistently for you. I turn off the ringer on the phone, as lovingly as possible tell my husband that I need some space, and close the bedroom door.

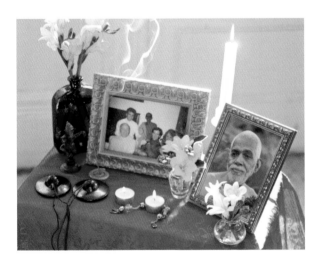

For how long should you meditate? When you're first learning, don't go for *length* but for *depth*. Start with 3 minutes, and work up to 15 minutes. Within that time, you'll probably include a few rounds of breathing. In the beginning, you might be meditating for only 5 minutes—and that's a great place to start.

PREPARING YOUR MIND AND BODY FOR MEDITATION

When you sit down to meditate, there are some steps you can take to lead yourself into it. Taking a few moments to prepare yourself can help you to enjoy your meditation and feel more successful.

1. SET YOUR INTENTION. Focus your awareness on the "cave of the heart," the center of your chest, midpoint between the breasts. Consciously set your intention to give yourself completely to the meditation time (even if it's just 2 minutes). Strengthen your determination with an affirmation: Yes, I can! Yes, I will! You can even look at yourself in the mirror when you do this. Look into your own eyes so that your affirmations are sent to a deeper level. I like to imagine you are making eye contact with your wisdom body, vijnana-maya-kosha.

2. ACKNOWLEDGE THE WITNESS SELF. Close your eyes and mouth gently. Slide your tongue behind the back of your front upper teeth. This relaxes your jaw. Direct your inner gaze toward

the cave of the heart. Shine the light of your attention into it. Here, the witness is said to dwell. Visit that sweet space for a few moments. Acknowledge sakshin, your loving witness companion upon your journey.

3. CHOOSE YOUR BREATHING. Select one of the breathing techniques that feels comfortable to you, such as Three-Part Breathing, Kapalabhati, or alternate nostril breathing from chapter 11, or Sipping Breath from chapter 15. Make sure you can practice it with ease and without much thought. Pranayama enhances your one-pointed concentration, calms the mind, oxygenates your blood, and energizes the body.

4. PREPARE THE BODY FOR MEDITATION. Sitting still for meditation is not as easy as it sounds. The bed-top yoga series below will make a big difference in your ability to sit (almost) quietly in meditation. It is a series of yoga postures you can do on your bed as soon as you wake up in the morning. It helps to prepare your body for the stillness of meditation. Your mind can only be still if your body is also still.

Bed-Top Yoga Series for Meditation

Bed-top yoga is a 10-minute preparation for your hips, knees, feet, and ankles. Each pose is comfortably held and quietly focused for approximately three to six long, slow breaths. You don't have to do all of the poses each time. You'll benefit even if you do a couple each day. I enjoy doing some or all of these moves most mornings. The stretches truly help my achy knees and back and keep my legs from falling asleep.

To get started, slide into the center of your bed (or ease down to the floor and onto your mat, if it's nearby). As you move from pose to pose, adjust your nightclothes to your comfort zone. Warm? Cool? Tight or loose? There are no rules. Just enjoy the yin moment—the warmth and security of pillows and blankets; nowhere to go, nothing to do. Newspapers will wait.

STARGAZING YOGODA

- Lie down on your back, knees bent and heels comfortably close to your seat, your feet apart. Place your head on a pillow and your hands behind your head. This is Stargazing position.

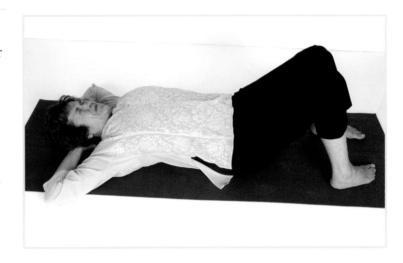

- Inhale slowly. Enjoyably and gently arch your spine, keeping your shoulders and hips on the bed. Release. Exhaling, press your lower back down.

- Repeat, but this time when you inhale and arch your spine, press your elbows back into the pillow. Squeeze your face and gently tense your chest, abdominals, and leg muscles. Hold the tension, then release. Exhale. Feel the sensations within your body. Repeat two or three times.

YAWN WITH AWARENESS

- Imagine a tiny vortex of energy beginning to swirl way in the back of your throat. Feel the spiral nudging the mouth to open. Lift your eyebrows and shoulders, and raise your arms over your head. Squeeze your eyes shut, dilating your nostrils and stretching the tight jaw "hinge."

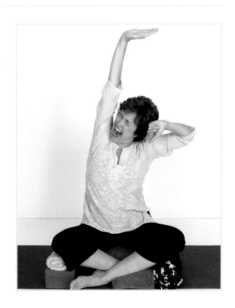

- Inhaling, your chest lifts, lungs expand, and the heart beats faster, sending a blast of energy to your brain. Exhaling, send this swirling spiral all the way down to your toes as you enjoyably stretch from side to side. Repeat. As you exhale, use a waking-up yawn sound.

KNEES TO CHEST

- First arrange the bedding so that you are warm and comfortable. I enjoy pulling the sheets up over my chest. Bring both knees to your chest, hands behind your thighs, knees open. Exhaling, draw knees and thighs to chest. Inhale and release slowly. Repeat six to eight times.

LYING DOWN TWIST

- Place your body in the center of your bed. With knees bent, lift your hips up and swish your hips 2 inches to the right. Drop your hips down, then drop both bent knees to the left. If you like, place pillows between and on either side of your knees for comfort (pillows not shown in photo). Now place your arms in a T position. Turning your head, look over your right shoulder. Enjoy these next few breaths. Inhale . . . nice long in-breath. Then slowly exhale, emphasize the exhalation, and pull the navel in firmly. Repeat this breath two or three times.

- Return spine to center, swish hips 2 inches to the left, and repeat with both knees to the right. Prop your knees, and look over your left shoulder. Repeat the emphasis on a long exhale.

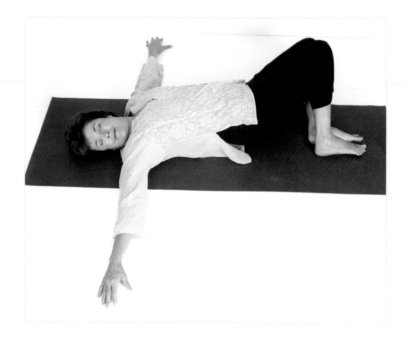

DANCING THE STAR

- Keep bedding across your upper body for warmth. Bend your knees, keeping them about 4 inches apart. Place your hands on your knees, keeping your arms straight. Now guide the knees into two separate circles, with your feet dangling. Open the knees to widen the circular motion. Breathing, enjoy the feeling of your hips waking up. Finally, open your knees as wide as possible. This is called Dancing the Star.

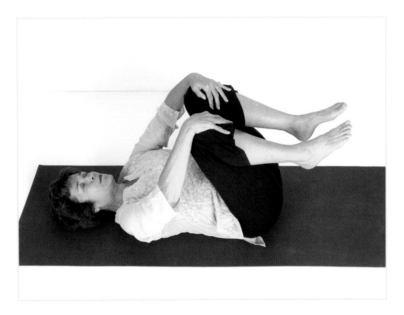

- Now repeat in the other direction, starting small and ending with large, wide circles. Hold for two or three breaths, with knees opened comfortably. Pause, and bring your knees together. Place your feet on the bed. Take two or three complete breaths.

Piriformus with Table / Cat / Cow

For more details of this important hip stretch, please refer to page 143.

- Lie faceup, knees bent, with a pillow behind your head. Place your right ankle on your left thigh, near the knee. The right ankle bone is well supported by your thigh. Reach your right arm between your legs and clasp your left hand, holding on to the left leg, as shown. If it is more comfortable, hold on to the back of your thigh or use a belt around the thigh.

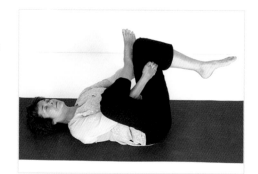

- Gently pull the folded left leg toward your left shoulder, keeping your back and hips down. Hold for two to three breaths. Close your eyes . . . observe the feeling of the stretch in your right leg. This is your piriformus lengthening.

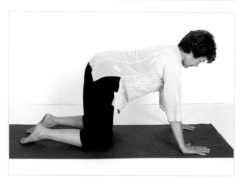

- Now do the three Rs. Your right ankle is pressed gently into your left leg, which in turn presses in toward your chest. Feel your right hip muscle tighten. Hold (Resist) for two or three breaths—about 6 seconds. Breathe in and Relax your whole body. Repeat. Slowly pull your folded left leg closer to your left armpit and ribs (Restretch). Hold for two or three breaths.

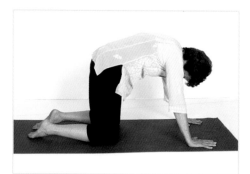

- Now come onto your hands and knees, into Table Pose.

- Exhaling, round your back into Cat Pose.

- Then, inhaling, drop your back into Cow Pose. Repeat for three or four breaths. Move smoothly from one breath into another. Stay in Table Pose as you move into the next few poses.

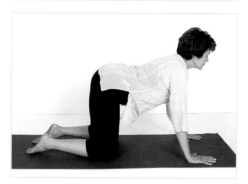

MECCA POSE

- While in Table Pose, place a pillow on the floor beneath your chest. Your knees are open. Turn your toes under and sit back comfortably toward your heels. Fold your arms and rest your forehead on them.

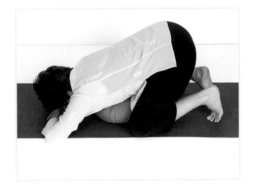

- Now stretch your arms out in front of you. Pause, and enjoy the stretch. Then "walk" your hands to the right and pause. Then walk your hands back to center. Now walk them to the left and pause. Feel which muscles are lengthening—enjoy it! Walk back to center.

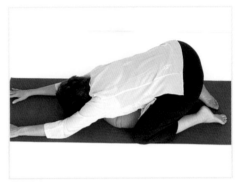

- Now place the tops of your feet to the floor and, again, gently press your hips back. Feel the toes stretch. Hold for two or three breaths. Sit up so you are sitting directly on top of your heels. Hold, then release. Now go right into Frog Pose.

FROG POSE

- Lie on your abdomen with your legs straight and your arms folded beneath your head. Bend your left knee, sliding it up comfortably close to your left armpit. You may place a pillow under your chest if it feels good. Take a moment to allow your hip and leg to sink into the surface.

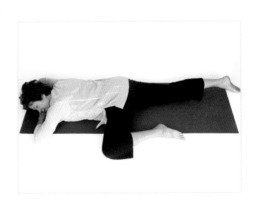

- Do the three Rs. Press the bent knee down into the bed. Hold (Resist) for two or three breaths. Inhale; Relax. Exhale, sink hips deeper (Restretch). Repeat on opposite side.

LEGS IN V POSE

- Sit in the center of your bed, and slide your legs as wide apart as is comfortable into a V, with no strain. Place lots of firm pillows in front of your chest. Then lean forward so your chin hangs over the ledge of pillows. Your neck is long. Place your arms on the insides of your legs and let your whole body go limp, allowing gravity to naturally and slowly lengthen your muscles. Hold for six breaths.

- Now do the three Rs. Build up a little resistance by pressing arms into legs, and legs into arms. Hold, remembering the three-R directions. Resist steadily and gently for 6 breaths. Relax; breathe in. Restretch, exhaling. Perhaps you now can widen the V a bit more. Slowly sit up.

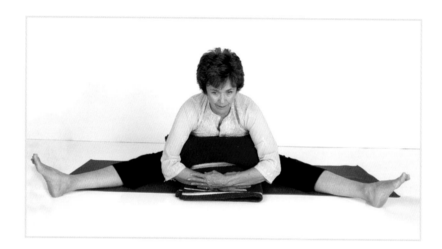

CHAPTER 15

TIME TO MEDITATE

"IF YOUR MIND WANDERS AWAY 57 TIMES, YOU MUST GENTLY AND WITHOUT EMOTION BRING IT BACK TO THE OBJECT OF MEDITATION 57 TIMES WITHOUT VEXATION OR IRRITATION. IF YOU GET UPSET OR IMPATIENT, YOU WILL LOSE YOUR MEDITATIVE STATE. EVENTUALLY THE MIND CATCHES ON AND REALIZES THAT IT IS FAR EASIER TO FIX ON AN OBJECT THAN TO CONTINUE WANDERING."

—*Goswami Kriyananda (Founder, Temple of Kriya Yoga)*

Are you skeptical of meditation? For some folks, the word "meditation" conjures up exotic images, something mysterious and not of this world. But it's really not all that mystifying. Meditation is simply the practice of bringing your body and mind into a deep state of calm. Most of us can admit that in our busy, often stressful lives, we could use some calm! I hope you'll at least give meditation a try. In this chapter, I've tried to include simple, specific instructions for a few different meditations.

As you do the meditations, remind yourself to be patient with the antics of your mind. Getting frustratred with your mind is like getting mad at traffic. The traffic doesn't care! The mind is going to wander off and play. This is its nature. No need to get annoyed when this happens. I find that I have to acknowledge, again and again, "Oops, my mind has wandered." Then matter-of-factly, without emotion, I bring it back to my chosen meditation. With time and detachment, the impulse of the mind to interfere and control is softened. What a blessing!

Let's start by getting into position for meditation.

POSITIONING FOR MEDITATION

I recommend you experiment with my technique for "pillow propping" your hips and knees. Find what feels comfortable to you.

Sit on a firm pillow, with your hips higher than your ankles. Slide one foot in front of the other. Use small pillows to support your ankles, larger ones to lift your knees. As you can see in the photo, my ankles are in a nice long line with my knees.

Place your hands comfortably in your lap. Draping a shawl across your shoulders feels good in meditation.

Once you've found the right position for you, it's time to meditate. Try any of the following techniques.

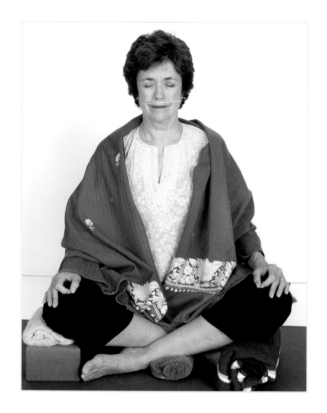

FOCUSED MEDITATION

This is a very basic approach to meditation and a good one to start with. My friend Larry Payne recommends it in his book *Yoga R$_x$*, and these instructions are his.

A favorite object of meditation is one's own breath. It's certainly convenient, and the yogis maintain it's a direct channel to your authentic self.

Sit comfortably, close your eyes, and begin to focus on your inhalation and your exhalation.

As you inhale through your nose, count to yourself, "One." Exhale. Then, on the next inhale, count, "Two," and so on. After each inhalation, try to hold your breath for one short beat before the exhalation. That short, quiet pause

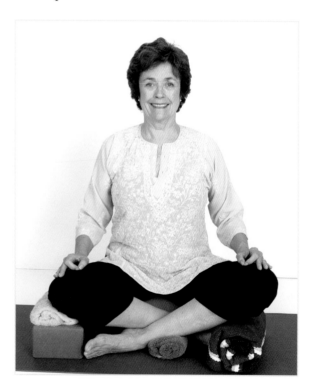

may serve as a doorway into meditation because at that point you are close to stillness.

How high can you count before you lose track completely? Be honest with yourself. Don't be shocked if you forget the count fairly quickly. Just go back to square one and start again. Keep trying until you can count straight through to 10; if you get to 10, go back and count to 10 again. Strengthening your ability to focus is like strengthening a muscle. The more you exercise your awareness, the stronger it gets.

WAVE OF BREATHING MEDITATION

"Inspiration" means to breathe in, to bring in something that comes from a higher place. Expiration is when the breath leaves the body. Watching the rhythm of the breath is an ancient, classic, relaxing way to engage the mind. Observing and listening to the waves of breath is like the enjoyment of listening to the waves of the great ocean rolling in and out.

Sitting, close your eyes. Observe your breath. Notice the rise and fall of your chest during everyday breathing. Changing nothing, breathe normally. Feel a oneness with all of creation, rich or poor, good or evil, as your breath flows in and out. Observe the coolness and warmth as the breath comes and goes. With the in-breath, your chest expands—your belly moves in and out. Simply watch the flow in and flow out, like the waves rolling onto shore . . . they roll in . . . and roll out.

The whole body pulsates in rhythm with the breath. Notice when the mind wanders away. Gently bring it back to the wave that flows in and out.

Listen for the sound the breath makes on its inward and outward journey. Breathe as it rolls in and out. Continue to be aware of the sound.

For a moment, tap into the place of peace, still and calm within you. Stillness of breath . . . even the sound of the waves float on stillness . . . stillness of mind . . . and stay a few moments longer . . . sense it as fully as you can.

Come out of meditation slowly. Reflect on the stillness within . . . write down any insights that might have come to you. Take the small oasis of calmness with you on into your day.

THE SIPPING BREATH WITH CONTENTMENT MEDITATION

The Sipping Breath is a pleasant, natural energizer. It's unique because you can do it on your back, sitting up, or on all fours (Table Pose or Frog Pose). It works well with the contentment meditation, but don't do Sipping Breath if you want to go to sleep, because it will wake you up!

Imagine your lungs are three separate compartments or rooms, and you are going to fill each space separately with vibrant, sparkling energy and life force. Begin sitting up tall, your spine long. Be at full attention without tension.

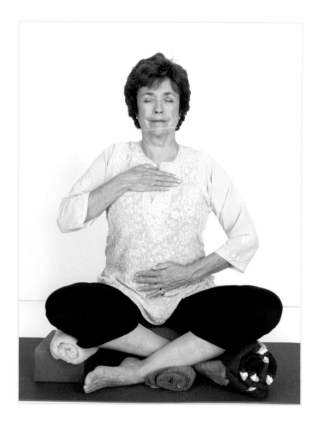

Take a moment to scan inside your mouth. Unlock your jaw; your tongue floats. Focus your one-pointed attention down to your belly. (Place your thumb on your navel if you want to find your belly.) This is the basement. Close your eyes; focus your attention down into this large, expansive room. Take three or four effortless sips of breath to fill the basement. Pause without exhaling. Focus awareness into the second room, your midchest and ribs. You may place your a hand on your chest if it helps you to focus there. Take three or four more little sips. Pause, still without exhaling. Now into the upper room; one or two little sips. Fill; pause.

Then exhale very, very slowly. Make it even and comfortable, all the way to the depths of your basement, gently pulling in muscles behind the navel area. Do it again. Keep your focus. Effortlessly fill the basement with three or four short sips . . . pause. Now fill the midchest with two or three short sips . . . pause. Now fill the upper room; short, effortless little sips. Pause at the ceiling of your upper room. Now, exhale nice and slowly, evenly.

After you've done a few rounds of Sipping Breath, pause. Now it's time to go into the contentment meditation. Close your eyes . . . dive inward. Listen to the stream of inner stillness. When a thought floats through to get your attention, turn it into a big log. Choose not to develop the thought. Watch the log float by, and return to listening to the stream of stillness. Do a few more rounds of Sipping Breath. Pause . . . dive inward. When thoughts arise (and they will), gently let them float on by.

Remember, meditation is effortless effort. The purpose is not really to accomplish something. It's simply a feeling of full attention without tension. You know how to relax. Scan your body for tension. Use the witness to observe any restlessness, such as tightness in the jaw or shoulders.

Consciously remain sitting for a few minutes longer to enjoy the quietude. This quietude is known as *santosha*, contentment. Smile; reconnect with your contentment, which contains the fullness, the beauty, and the sweetness of life. It has never left you.

There is nothing more to do, nothing more to seek. Feel it. Breathe around its sweetness. Keep it with you as you go through your day.

SHHH BREATHING

This is a sweet little breath I do when I and my witness can see some old repetitious thoughts begin to resurface, disrupting my meditation time or as I walk through life.

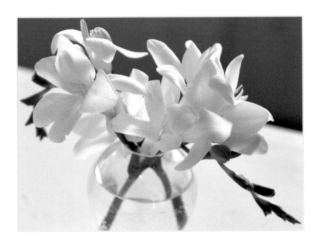

Without anger or criticism, look at the thought very much as you would a beloved crying baby that needs attention. I tenderly gather the thought to my chest and say aloud three or four times, *Shhh . . . Shhh . . . Shhh . . .* with all the tenderness I can muster. The mind, like a restless infant, seems to smile, soften, and calm down, and I can continue enjoying the stillness of meditation.

DEVELOPING YOUR WISDOM BODY TAKES TIME

As meditation and relaxation practice deepens, your ability to connect with your wise inner guidance is enhanced. You are able to stand back and take an expanded view of life situations. You can recognize your own core beliefs, the ones that guide your daily behavior, and learn to defuse them if they're outdated or inaccurate. Even painful life events can be viewed in an objective and calm manner.

Be patient and of good cheer. As your vijnana-maya-kosha grows more balanced and strong, your clarity of judgment, increased willpower, and greater intuitive insight will strengthen as well.

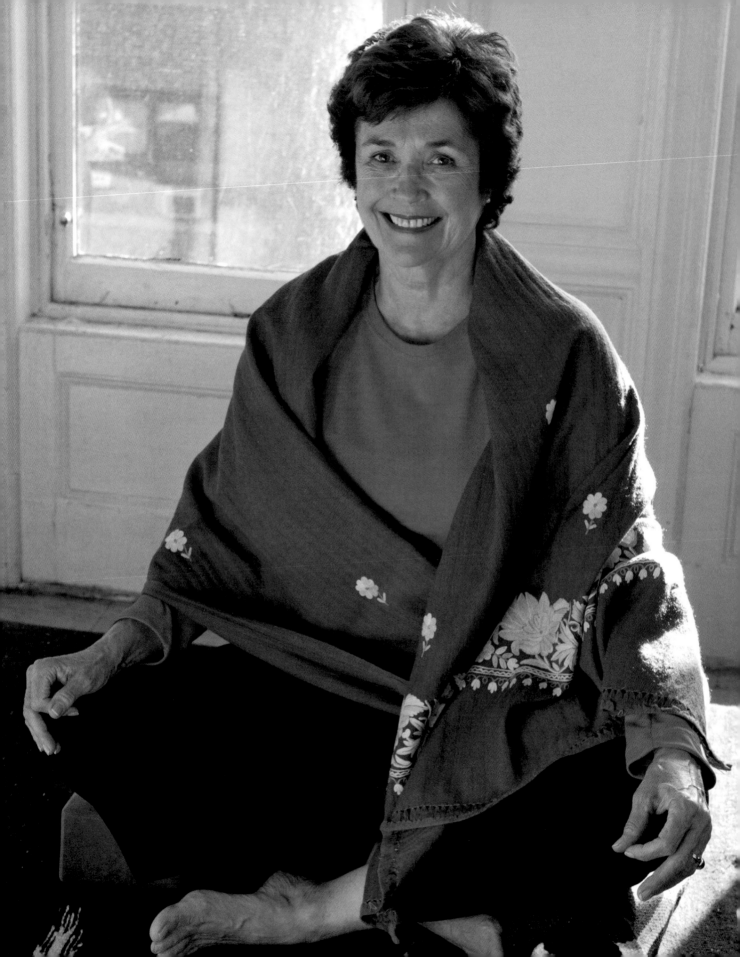

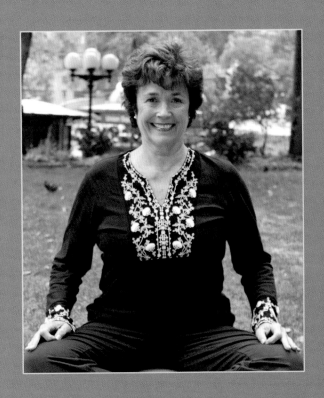

PART SEVEN

ANANDA-MAYA-KOSHA

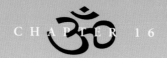

CHAPTER 16

YOUR BLISS BODY

> "WHAT IS A GENUINE MYSTERY? A SMILE ORIGINATING IN
> THE DEPTHS OF THE SOUL. THAT IS A MYSTERY."
> —*Gitta Mallasz,* Talking with Angels

Thus far we've discussed the first four koshas—our physical, energy, emotional, and wisdom bodies. It helps to visualize them as sheaths, one on top of the other, with the first sheath, the physical body, on the outside, and the others layered successively within. We now come to the deepest, innermost layer, the fifth sheath, known as *ananda-maya-kosha. Ananda* is a Sanskrit word that major spiritual teachers say is truly impossible to translate. It is often called "the bliss body." Feelings (not to be confused with emotions) such as stillness, love, peace, ease, and contentment are often used to describe the ananda state. Ananda is said to be the most balanced "living wisdom" a human being can experience. My question is: If it's so darn blissful, wise, and balanced, why isn't it easier for you and me to experience?

Well, you probably have experienced glimpses but just never labeled them as such. Remember the stillness you felt gazing as a sunset? No words . . . just deep stillness and beauty. The wonder you felt looking into the eyes of a new-born baby or listening to magnificent music? For me, it's the silent awe and delight I felt as I marveled at Michelangelo's *David* in Florence, Italy.

Separation from ananda, the bliss body, amounts to a painful denial of our true nature. The ananda-maya-kosha is extremely important in yoga because it is the final and thinnest veil that stands between ordinary awareness and our High Self. Karen Armstrong, in her book *A History of God,* called it a God Hole or God Space that possibly was easily accessible to primitive humans. Millions of years later, that veiled space has clouded over, causing a disconnect from spirit, our most powerful source of healing.

My own ananda-maya-kosha, my God Space, was awakened with a jolt. I'd like to share the story with you.

I sat alone on the bow of our small boat early in the morning fog. My husband, Bob, deftly guided us around the shrouded buoys floating in Long Island Sound. I closed my eyes, enjoying the sounds of the foghorn and the peace in floating securely homeward.

In that relaxed, no-thought moment, I suddenly dropped inward and could feel a deep stirring inside my chest. The stirring could be best described as a pressure, like a big thumb was pressing from the inside out . . . and with that pressure came a longing. Behind the pressure were blue and red flickering flames, like a deep, burning furnace emanating wave after wave of longing and bliss. I thought my longing meant I was to leave my home, my children, everything, and go live in an ashram or convent, dedicating my life to the blissful, longing adoration of God.

Totally confused by the indescribable experience and feelings, I took them to the only person who would understand: my spiritual teacher, Swami Chidananda, then residing at the Sivananda Yoga Center in Val Morin, Quebec, Canada.

Tearfully, I told the swami of my experience and the angst it had caused. He was quiet. Then he asked me, "Did it feel like a thumb pressing from the inside of your chest out?" I nodded. He told me quietly, "Lilias, you have been called by God, but you were called after your marriage, not before." What he suggested was that within my home, with husband, two boys, and a golden retriever, I would find all that I would ever need to stay connected to the spiritual heart and God Space.

Twenty years have passed since that boat ride on foggy Long Island Sound. My brief glimpse into a spiritual realm beyond my comprehension caused me to begin thinking differently about certain words like "bliss" and especially "love." I had experienced a deeper, bigger aspect of love, and even though I didn't really understand it, I knew love was much more than the treacle-like, syrupy sweet emotion we associate with hearts and flowers. It had something to do with God and the universe and how we're all connected. Little did I know that 2 decades later my ananda-maya-kosha would be jolted again. It was time to learn more.

To be asked to teach hatha yoga within a college was a dream come true—and at the Cincinnati Conservatory of Music, no less! I was thrilled to be teaching these young, talented musicians. Being invited to a college made me feel as though a deeper level of respect and acceptance of yoga had finally arrived.

But unfortunate worries arrived as well: "What if no one comes? What if I'm not perfect? What exotic yoga postures shall I teach them? Wisdom, that's what they need." I pored over my philosophy books and decided to quote the wise, hip rebel philosopher J. Krishnamurti: "If you begin to understand what you are, without trying to change it, then what you are undergoes a transformation."

For 2 weeks, the angst and planning continued. Finally my big morning arrived. Getting ready for class, as I stood half-dressed, balancing on one foot, putting on my black tights, my worried inner talking continued. "What if no one comes? What if they don't like me? What shall I say? What shall I do?"

From nowhere, yet everywhere, a voice boomed, *"Sit down."* Speechless, my bottom hit the floor. My mind wiped clean, and I was silent. I listened as the voice told me, *"Just love them."* Weakly, the worries tried to struggle to the surface. Again the voice repeated, *"Just love them."*

Seamless, silent impressions, not words, began to penetrate my being. Just love them . . . the real you is love . . . be that love . . . there is absolutely nothing more important, no words, no techniques . . . love is within the essence of all postures and breathing, hidden in every word. Love is within all your doings. You don't have to "say" anything. Just *be.* Be the awareness of the love that passes all understanding.

Charged with the wondrous high voltage of love's electricity, I went to the Cincinnati Conservatory. I forgot to read the Krishnamurti quote and gave a simple class. The students went easily into relaxation. Afterward, I watched the students sit up slowly. Some came over to talk, a little stunned by their depth of relaxation. Apparently they too had received some of the electrical charge.

It's taken years and maturity to understand what transpired that day and to more deeply appreciate the words of J. Krishnamurti. Sometimes we must get a little lost to become found. There is nowhere to go . . . nowhere to search, nothing to grasp or change . . . no more looking for love in all the wrong places. It's all within. Welcome home!

To this day, I will tell you I'm not an expert on this subject of finding the love, the bliss, within. But my experience has shown me that it wasn't until midlife that I was able to focus on intentionally starting to pursue this aspect of myself, uncovering the fifth kosha. As we spend time and interest nourishing peace and bliss within, it softens the veil, allowing us to become ever closer to our deepest wellspring of what the mystics call "living wisdom" or "bliss."

As you move into the following sections in which I've given specific ways to connect with your bliss body, take your time. Remember, the joy is in the journey. Your bliss is closer than you can imagine—within your own genuine smile, the sweetness of Caring Breath, and even with a heart-centered Lunge Pose. And in the next chapter, we'll look at one more powerful way to connect with the bliss body—through getting in touch with our gratitude.

CONNECTING WITH YOUR BLISS BODY

A ray of bliss is as close to you and as available as your own human smile. A smile is a restorative gift that radiates joy and healing, not only from the heart of the smiler, but also to the smiled upon.

I experienced this firsthand. I was standing alone by the bed of my mother-in-law as she lay dying. I loved her dearly, and it was my first time dealing with death. A nurse walked into the room. I had never met her before, but she listened quietly as I poured out my grief. I do not recall her words, but I do remember the understanding and healing energy she transmitted to me with her sweet smile. I was ready to cope with whatever was to come.

Chinese masters regard emotions such as fear, worry, anger, and sadness as neither bad nor good, just low-grade energy. This stressful energy drains our life force, causing tension and stress on organs, and instability of the mind. But a true, genuine smile originates in your spiritual heart. It produces a high-grade, healing energy, which is easily "transmitted" to internal organs, glands, bone marrow, and the nervous system. Equally important, anyone can transmit this force to another person. The sender will benefit from the exchange as much as the receiver will.

Today, the human smile is the subject of study. After two decades of research, Paul Ekman, Ph.D., a psychologist at the University of California at San Francisco, concluded there are 18 types of smiles, but only one is the true smile that produces positive emotional benefits. A polite smile, grin-and-bear-it grimace, or make-nice smile will not give you the psychological lift that comes with a genuine smile of enjoyment. The following feelings have been associated with a genuine smile that can awaken your bliss body: thankfulness, gratitude, appreciation, delight, awe, amazement, and longing (to name a few). You've experienced all of them.

Dr. Ekman's research shows that we can voluntarily "create" this true smile and tap into its feel-good healing benefits. Try it now. Begin by focusing your attention on your lips. Feel the length of your lips . . . let the corners curl up . . . feel your cheeks raise and activate the little laugh lines around your eyes. Your lips are softly closed. This is the outer beginning to your "inner smile."

Traditionally, Taoist masters from the 6th century B.C. considered the inner smile so precious and sacred that they whispered it in secret, passing the confidence on only to those students deemed worthy of and ready for the information. The sages' high esteem for the gesture was based on their observation that the most accessible and immediate form of bliss energy was in a sincere smile. In a moment, you'll take one of the feelings associated with a genuine smile with you into a wonderful relaxation-meditation called the inner smile. From this moment on, let go . . . release all expectations for the outcome of this practice.

Inner Smile Relaxation

I have taught this exercise for many years in classes and workshops. I've particularly enjoyed teaching it to the participants of Dr. Dean Ornish's retreats featuring his Program for Reversing Heart Disease.

Preparation: Choose a quiet spot. Take the phone off the hook. Later on, you will be able to practice inner smile anytime and anywhere. For today, close the door, stay warm, and loosen your belt. Remove your glasses and watch. Sit or lie down. Be comfortable. Breathe nor-

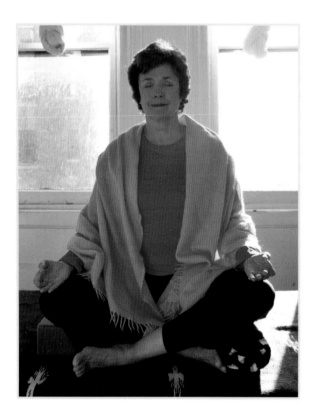

mally . . . then a few long, smooth exhales. Close your eyes . . . focus your attention to the inside of your mouth. Slide your tongue close to your front upper teeth. Feel little lines of cares and worries begin to melt away. Daydream . . . let an image of great beauty come to you. Perhaps it's someone you love. Let that smiling, sweet energy fill your mouth . . . softening your jaw. Feel the length of your lips . . . let the corners of your lips turn up . . . enough to raise your cheek muscles and little laugh lines.

Now take your smiling energy, like a beam of light, up into your left eye, then your right eye . . . left ear and then right ear . . . left brain and then right brain . . . return to your mouth. Recharge your smile with an image of great beauty . . . corners of your lips turned up . . . smile down into your neck and throat . . . Your neck is jammed with activity. Your smiling energy opens into your throat. Tensions melt away.

Let that smiling energy flow into your heart . . . a little left of the center of your chest . . . the heart is the seat of compassion . . . honest respect. Let your smiling energy fill your heart with joy. Thank your heart for its constant work. Feel it open and relax as it works with more ease.

Now radiate this smiling, thankful energy from your heart into your lungs. Thank your lungs for their wonderful work in supplying oxygen to your whole body. Feel them soften, become spongier and moist. Send the light of your smile deeply into your lungs. Smile your sadness and depression away. Fill the lungs with smiling gratefulness, from the heart. Now let it flow down into the liver.

Smile into your liver . . . the right side, beneath your rib cage . . . Thank it for marvelous work in digestion and detoxifying harmful substances. Feel it soften and grow moist. Smile again, deep into your liver. See any anger or hot temper in the liver. Smile them away. Let the joyfulness and gratitude induce the warmth of kindness to flow.

Smile your energy into your kidneys . . . just below your rib cage above each hip. Thank them for their work of filtering waste products and maintaining water balance . . . Feel them grow cool, fresh, and clean . . . As you smile deeper into your kidneys, see and feel if any fear resides inside . . . Smile your warm thanks, grateful, kindly energy into the kidneys . . . Melt your fears away. Let gentleness . . . the nature of the kidneys . . . come out . . . into all other organs, bones, immune system of the body . . . .

If you have someplace in your body that needs a little extra love today, smile into that discomfort or uneasiness. Spend time smiling into any sick parts of your body. Talk to them. Visualize them getting softer . . . more open . . . their color changing from dark to light . . . .

Now . . . visualize the organs of your body . . . smiling at you . . . (long pause).

Return to your mouth. For one last time . . . smile up into your brain . . . Feel your good friend the brain . . . smiling down on you . . . (long pause). Now rest . . . let all the technique go . . . dissolve . . . into clear blue sky of awareness . . . and rest . . . rest, in this timeless moment.

Practice inner smile in a shortened version each day as you wake up. In sending love throughout your body, you become more loving to others and more effective in your work. If you have a short time, take a few minutes to radiate the smile throughout your body. Practice at times of stress, anger, fear, impatience, and other draining, low-grade emotions.

CARING BREATH

Caring Breath is aptly named: arm and head movements combine with a relaxing breathing technique, directing your sweet, caring energy toward yourself. When you bow your head, your thoughts immediately quiet down.

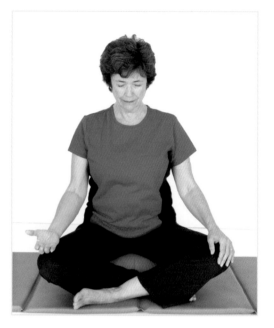

- Sit comfortably. Place your hands on your knees, with your right palm up, left palm down. Take a few breaths.

- Bow your head. Inhaling, raise your right forearm and your head. Pause.

- Exhaling, turn your head comfortably to your left and bring your right hand to the left side of your chest. Pause.

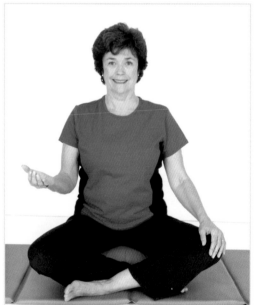

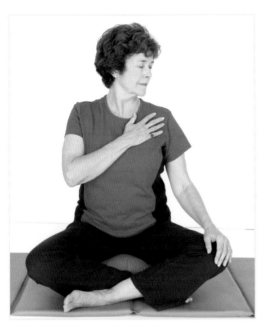

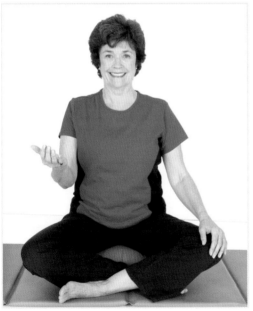

- Inhaling, slowly bring your head and forearm to the front, as you did in the second step. Pause.

- Exhaling, bow your head and lower your right arm. Pause for 4 seconds. Soften your face and eyes.

- Continue inhaling and exhaling four or five more times, emphasizing the pause.

- Now raise your head and left arm, turning to your right and bringing your left hand to the right side of your chest.

- Continue alternating arms, and emphasize the pause. Practice three to five times on each side. Then sit quietly, eyes relaxed, hands settled comfortably in your lap or on your knees. Let a smile come to your lips. Focus your attention deeply inward. Feel nurtured, soothed, and cared for. Sit for a few more minutes, enjoying the quiet.

THE HEART LUNGE

Men and women from all spiritual and religious traditions use their hands and feet as a way to "anchor" themselves, bringing deeper meaning and intention to the heart of prayer. There is a saying, "My feet were praying," which seems to mean you can use your whole body to open your heart center. Actions, thoughts, and movements in yoga practice can be an expression of the heart. We don't just think our prayers . . . but can feel them deeply in the body. With the Heart Lunge, we find a way to feel and express the idea, "I give and receive love today."

Join me now. Put your thinking aside, close your eyes, extend your hands outward, palms up in the gesture of giving. Take a moment to welcome the divine into your life, and give away your hands in service to the source of all life.

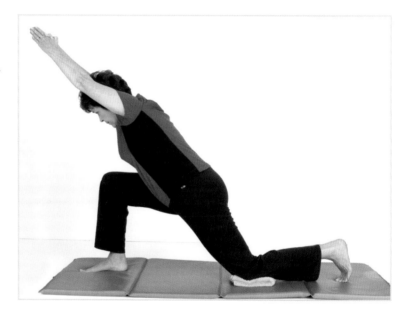

- Begin in a modified Lunge Pose. Your back knee is aligned under its hip, and your front knee is over its ankle. The back knee stays on the mat or a folded towel. Lift up your heart until your spine is vertical.

- Place the palms of your hands together, in the center of your chest (in the familiar "praying position.") Pause here, letting your hands say, "I welcome the divinity within." Inwardly feel, "I want to know you!"

- Now extend your arms out to form a T, palms up in the gesture of giving. Then arch your spine, pull your arms back, and open your chest. Look up, smile, and lift up your heart. Breathe. Give your heart away today. Offer it to your family, to those in need, to all beings. No matter how much love you give away, there is always plenty for all. Hold for two or three breaths.

● While still in the modified Lunge position, lean forward, with your rib cage over your forward thigh. Slowly extend both arms forward until they are straight up near your ears (as in the photo on the previous page). Continuing to reach out in front of you, press your palms together, cross your thumbs, and bow your head in gratefulness. Hold for two breaths.

● Return to the first step, but this time give yourself a hug. Elbows cross your chest . . . lift your elbows in line with your throat . . . hands hold on to shoulders (like you did in Garuda I). Pause . . . ask yourself, what does it feel like to receive love? Is it easier for me to give love than to receive it? Do I feel self-conscious hugging myself? Let any self-conscious feelings melt away. Hold the nurturing feelings of the hug for two or three breaths.

● Look up . . . then fling your arms open wide, and give away your love. Open your chest . . . arch your spine . . . go deeper into Heart Lunge. Your forward knee slides back an inch. Continue to breathe; hold 3 or 4 seconds. Release the pose. Bring both knees to the mat for Child's Pose . . . forehead to floor . . . reach back with two fists and tap, tap, tap the lower back to release any muscle tightness. Rest.

Absorb Heart Lunge into your body. Repeat the above steps on the opposite leg.

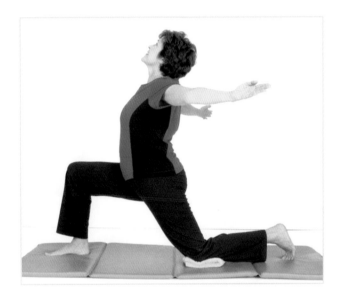

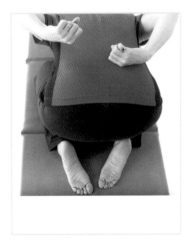

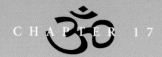
THE POWER OF GRATITUDE

"GRATITUDE IS THE HEART'S MEMORY."
—French proverb

As years have gone by, I look forward more and more to Thanksgiving Day, that traditional holiday when our whole family can gather together and express gratitude and thankfulness for our lives.

As part of my yoga practice, I've always tried to incorporate gratitude and thankfulness into my everyday life. It's important for me to take time to express gratefulness for my loving husband and appreciation for my two grown sons and their wives, who are amazing, caring, and thoughtful parents. I cherish and value my friends and try to take time during a busy day to make a call or jot a note. I remind myself of how fortunate I am to have yoga and spiritual teachers in my life, and of how much they've given me.

To some degree, we all need to break away from the hardened heart. A frosty "cave of the heart" produces a cold attitude toward everyone and everything. Warming up your light of appreciation and gratitude can have a positive impact on your health and, best of all, melt away grumpiness.

Intriguing scientific studies show what yogis have known intuitively for years: dwelling on what has gone wrong, past grievances, and old frustrations creates a nasty energy that affects your health. There are medically sound connections between positive emotions such as gratitude and a strong, efficient heart; vigorous immune and hormonal systems; and healthy blood pressure.

HARNESS THE HEALING POWER OF GRATITUDE

Because of the health benefits, I'd like to share with you some time-honored techniques I've learned to convert negative thoughts and feelings into positive expressions of gratitude and appreciation. They include affirmations, keeping a journal, meditating, and breathing. You do not have to use all at once. Simply choose one that feels most appropriate for you and incorporate it into your life.

Affirmations

Affirmations provide you with positive statements to replace negative messages that undermine your health. They replace the old, crabby thinking with thoughts that make you feel good.

Affirmation is a process also referred to as "auto suggestion," which takes a powerful word or phrase and continually repeats it. It is not a mantra, however. (I purposely have not mentioned the power of mantras in this book. Mantras have a deep effect on the human mind. It is a subject for the true experts to write about. I hope you take the time to read about mantras from my list of recommended readings on meditation, adding this knowledge to your personal practice.)

Here are some affirmations of gratitude and appreciation:

Today I am thankful for all that is positive in my life.

I am grateful to all the people who support and nurture me.

I appreciate my family, friends, and coworkers.

I appreciate myself as a unique, wonderful, and worthy person.

I appreciate my body's ability to heal as well as its continued health.

Feel free to make up any of your own. I have given you space for reflection on page 137.

Well-known yoga guru and author Sri Goswami Kriyananda, of the Temple of Kriya Yoga in Chicago, suggests that you occasionally use the following: "Everyday in every way, I am becoming more and more content." Using the words "I am becoming" acknowledges the moments when you are not content and reaffirms that, even though you may not be content at this moment, you will be content soon and with each passing hour.

It is most effective to use these affirmations at night before falling asleep and again first thing in the morning.

Keeping a Gratitude Journal

I continue to enjoy journaling as a way to express feelings of appreciation. In her book *Simple Abundance*, author Sarah Ban Breathnach talks about a gratitude journal. Writing down at least five things each day that you are thankful for helps you focus on what is going right in your life rather than what is going wrong. Keeping a little journal really has worked for me. They are also very interesting to read, sometimes even years later.

Here are a few thoughts to keep in mind:

▶ Select any kind of journal: a spiral notebook, loose-leaf binder, or bound book.

▶ Make an appointment with yourself and your friend, the witness, to meet with your journal a few minutes each day.

▶ Find a calm, safe place where you can write freely without disturbances.

▶ Do not worry about spelling, punctuation, or grammar.

▶ Refrain from censoring yourself as you write. The emotions, observations, and feelings written down are neither good nor bad. Once on paper, throw them out if you choose to. The important thing is to get them out.

▶ Finally, be honest, be real . . . be yourself!

Meditation on Gratitude

Close your eyes and ask yourself, "Where do I feel thankfulness in my body?" This is a question worth repeating. Pause a moment. Feel inside your body the feeling of gratitude. Now, place your hand on that place. Chances are your hand is on your chest. Loving emotions such as thankfulness radiate from the center of your chest—not your big toe! By focusing your attention on the feeling, you will intensify and experience for yourself this sweet, healing heart energy.

Entering the Cave of Your Heart

Sit comfortably . . . do four to six rounds of Caring Breath. Remember, as you read the following, to go slowly.

Close your eyes . . . hands resting in your lap . . . feel where your eyelids touch.

Focus your attention, your inner gaze, downward, away from the thought factory and into the center of your chest. Inhale and exhale slowly and easily. Enter the cave of your heart. Imagine you are lighting a candle and place it inside the cave . . . see its nurturing glow illuminating the darkness.

Visualize filling your cave heart with feelings of gratitude and appreciation. Feel the area of your heart glow with warm, loving emotions. The cave fills with the soft, golden light of grateful thanks.

Now, radiate your gratitude and appreciation to everyone who has helped and nurtured you, known and unknown . . . your family . . . friends . . . beloved pets . . . co-workers . . . your community.

Sit for a few more moments . . . enjoy the feeling of contentment . . . enjoy the quiet . . . the calm . . . the peace you have created within yourself.

To close, recall the candle . . . each time it goes out, the flame can be relit. If you would like, take your portable alter that is the cave of your heart with you into your day.

WRITE YOUR OWN AFFIRMATIONS

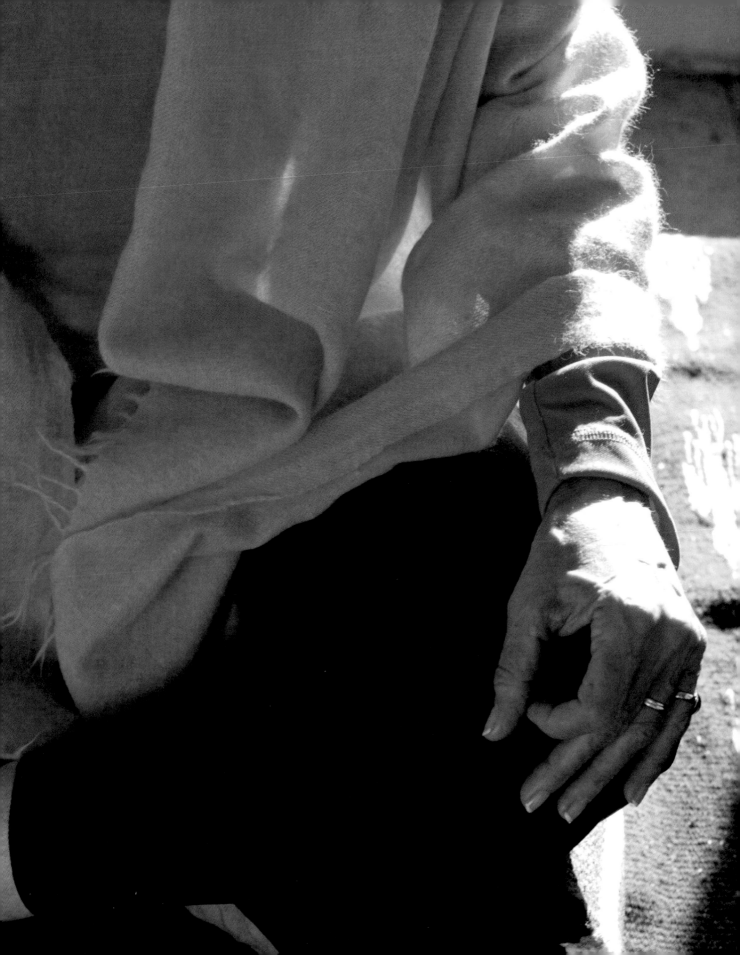

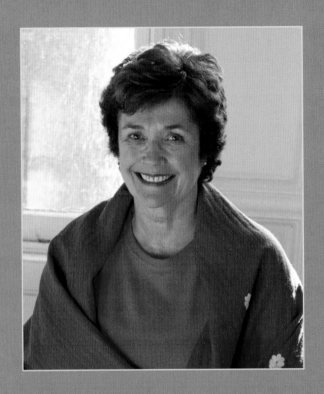

PART EIGHT

ATHA YOGA ANU
SHA SA NAM

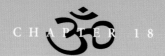

CHAPTER 18

YOGA POSTURES
FOR A DESERT ISLAND

Everything I've written in this book has brought you to this place of readiness. It is time to *practice yoga*. There are hundreds of yoga postures, plus hundreds more variations that keep postures interesting, but I have chosen only 44 of my favorite postures. I like to call them my "yoga postures for a desert island" because if I could only do a few, these are the ones I would choose.

I've grouped the postures in a way that makes sense according to how they are practiced—seated, lying on your back, standing, and so on. You can do them in this order, but you don't have to. In chapter 20, I offer some suggested routines, but feel free to make up your own.

Please, I encourage you to be creative. If there is a posture that you love but is not mentioned in this book, you can look at it with my yin approach. Pull the pose apart, warm up, and strengthen all the "pieces." Could using the three Rs help the comfort and flow of the pose? Above all, remember to breathe.

Throughout the postures, you'll see references to various yoga props. These are used to assist you in the pose, such as for leverage, increased stretch, or comfort. I often refer to "blocks," but

you can always use a large book instead. Yoga belts are handy, but I've used my husband's old neckties for years. A yoga mat is important, and many are available, but I especially recommend the Lili-Pad yoga mat, because I helped design it and I think it's perfect! Please refer to Appendix A for more information on props.

CHOOSING POSTURES

Every posture is not for everybody. Never feel you are a failure if you cannot master certain positions, even after years of practice. Start from where you are today. Keep your attitude positive. Yoga is much more than exercise. As you have read, it affects your entire self on many levels.

FIVE STEPS TO EACH ASANA (POSTURE)

THESE FIVE STEPS EQUAL ONE HARMONIOUS WHOLE—which is one great difference between doing calisthenics, Pilates, and yoga.

1. Attune yourself to the posture. Visualize your body going through the motion. Every posture feels different, the way Monday feels different from Friday. Feel for the difference.
2. As you come to know the posture, flow smoothly into and out of the pose. Breath and body move in harmony and awareness.
3. We usually hold for a few seconds at the end of a pose. Holding does not mean you are encased in cement. In the hold, you can move in increments to deepen the stretch. Concentration and endurance are also strengthened. Agitation is released.
4. Sweep out of each pose as beautifully as you went into it. Bring the posture to a close in your mind and body.
5. Relaxation is the final step. Here energies are balanced and emotions are quieted. Reconnect with stillness.

Right Side or Left Side?

I often begin with my right side to keep myself organized as to what I am doing in my own practice or while teaching. You'll find that one side is more difficult than the other in certain poses. The difficult, tight side indicates the side that is lacking. It is here that energy can be directed to strengthen your being. I highly recommend repeating the asana (posture) on the side that is tighter or more difficult to do.

Getting Motivated to Practice

"I don't have time to practice."

"I'm too busy."

I hear these excuses the most often. How many times have I listened to dynamic and successful people explain to me why they are unable to take time out of their busy days to focus on their healing journey? I can't even begin to guess, but here are some tricks that have helped me.

1. Morning is usually better for a 20-minute or longer practice to set up my day. (I, too, make up excuses!) For others, 20 minutes in the evening works better. If you need help getting motivated, try following a video. On the weekend, if you have more time, give yourself a nice 1-hour "work-in."
2. Place simple reminders around for you to see. Lay out your exercise clothes the night before. Keep your yoga mat rolled up but in plain view. Play some inspiring music; this *really* helps me.
3. Start with warming up. It will make your practice more pleasant and effective.
4. Write the word "Breathe," and post it in your car, on the phone, and mirror. One of my friends put BREATHE on his screen saver. It reminds him . . . to remember . . . to breathe!

In a Pinch

What causes muscle cramps? Some say cramping is a sign of fatigue. Others blame it on loss of sodium or potassium in the body. A third possibility is that cramps result from dehydration. Yet another explanation is that when muscles sustain continual tightness, they never get a chance to relax, and this leads to cramping. Whatever the cause, cramping is painful!

Here are a few precautions for cramp prevention:

▶ Stretch your legs before bed.
▶ Keep your muscles warm.
▶ Stay well hydrated.
▶ Massage, tap, or hit a muscle as soon as it cramps.

Lastly, here is my "pinch cure" for muscle cramps: Pinch the skin between your upper lip and below your nose. Hold for 20 seconds. I've tried it often and it works!

Yoga Buzzwords

Here are some terms that I often use in my posture descriptions.

BUCKLE UP SEAT BELT: Refers to the muscles behind your belly/navel area, also known as core abdominals, that hold and support your back and abdomen.

CLOSE THE GATES OF THE SHOULDERS: Refers to your scapulae, which close when you do Chest Expander. A vital piece of Half Shoulderstand, Bridge Pose, and other poses.

LIFT THE EYES OF THE HEART: Explanation, pictures, and breathing directions are on page 88.

Atha Yoga Anu Sha Sa Nam. And now we begin.

TABLE POSE (*MAJARIASANA*) WITH CAT, COW, AND SMILE

BENEFITS: *This pose flexes and extends your lower back, helps relieve symptoms of backache, and massages your internal organs.*

- Start in Table Pose, on your hands and knees. Relax your head so you're either comfortably looking up or naturally looking down. Your knees are hip-width apart, and your hands are below your shoulders. Elbows are straight, but not locked.

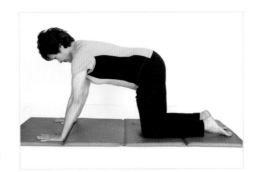

- Exhaling, round your back like an angry cat, and look at the floor.

- Inhaling, slowly look up to the ceiling. Drop your lower back in a reverse curve to form a little valley (or an old cow). Then alternate Cat and Cow six to eight times, in rhythm with your breathing.

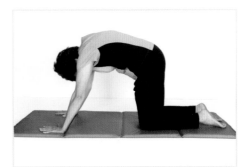

- Now walk your feet to the left. Look over your left shoulder to see your feet. Feel the enjoyable stretch on the right side of your body, which forms a "smile." Hold this smile for two or three breaths. Then walk your feet to the right and repeat the smile on the opposite side.

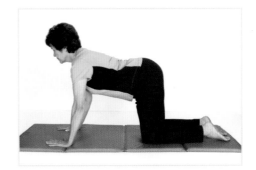

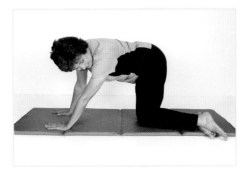

FLYING SUNBIRD (*CHAKRAVAKASANA*)

BENEFITS: *Flying Sunbird, a variation of Cat and Cow Pose, is a balance pose that strengthens both sides, the front, and the back of the body. Strengthens your "wobble" muscle. Builds concentration and confidence.*

USE THE FOLLOWING WARMUP:

Cat and Cow Pose (page 143)

LEVEL ONE

- While in Table Pose, remind yourself to be light on your wrists, not lock elbows, and buckle up seat belt muscles. Slowly straighten and raise your right leg, no higher than the level of your back. Gaze to the floor. Now, begin to shake your right leg. Become the mythical sunbird, shaking out its beautiful plumage. As you shake the leg, exhale with a long "ahhh" sound. This is not only fun and energizing but the long "ahhh" purges the lungs, and the shaking increases circulation to the leg, hopefully preventing leg cramps. (See page 142 for my tips for relieving leg cramps.) Repeat on the opposite side, and then rest in Child's Pose (page 164) for 1 minute.

LEVEL TWO

- Return to Table Pose. Inhaling, raise your right leg, then raise your left arm straight, close to your ear, palm down . . . and hold as you balance . . . for three or four breaths. Remember to be light on your right wrist. Gaze to the floor. Repeat on the opposite side, then rest in Child's Pose 1 minute.

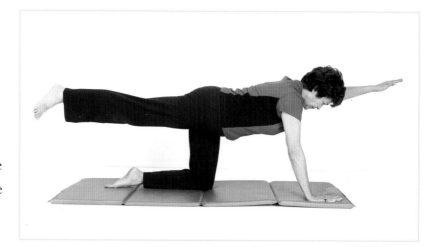

LEVEL THREE

- Now it's time for the sunbird to fly. Take it slowly—it looks simple, but a great number of muscles coordinate this simple move. Beginning in level two, lower your left arm and right leg a few inches . . . then lift them a few inches . . . slowly down and up. Continue "flying" four to six times, gazing to the floor. Check out your seat belt, keep your neck long, and remember to breathe! Repeat on the opposite side, then relax and rest in Child's Pose.

- Variation: Lift the same-side arm and leg together 8 to 10 times.

PIGEON PUSHUP (*KAPOTASANA*)

BENEFITS: *Warms and strengthens upper body and arms.*

- Sit comfortably and bend your knees, so your feet go toward your left and you're "sitting" on your right hip. With your knees still bent, gently pull your left thigh back to a comfortable place, and adjust your right leg so that your right foot is in front of your body. You may place a cushion or blanket beneath your right hip if you are stiff.

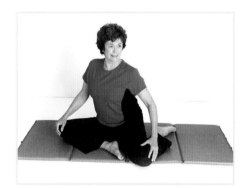

- Turn your chest to the right and place your hands shoulder-width apart on the floor. Your neck is long, in line with your spine. Exhaling, bend your elbows out to the sides and lower your chest and face toward the floor. Use seat-belt muscles for support. Breathe in . . . then on the exhale, press your palms into floor, as you pushup . . . repeat the pushup ten times, then repeat on the opposite side.

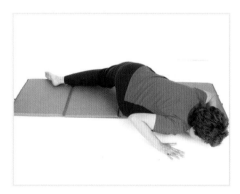

PIGEON I POSE: BENT KNEES

- Start in the beginning position for Pigeon Pushup. Turn your chest to the right, and place your hands on either side of your right bent knee. Lean forward, placing your elbows to the floor. Hold this stretch for two or three breaths, feeling your hips and back lengthen.

USE THE FOLLOWING WARMUPS:

Pigeon Pushup (page 145)

Table Pose with Cat and Cow (page 143)

Little Mermaid Series (pages 72–73)

Salutation to the Hips, all or part (page 216)

- The three Rs are very effective at this point, making Pigeon I Pose more comfortable and easier to hold. Gently press your forearms and your right thigh into the mat. Resist . . . holding the resistance for or four breaths . . . Relax . . . breathe in . . . and Restretch. Repeat . . . perhaps going deeper into Pigeon I.

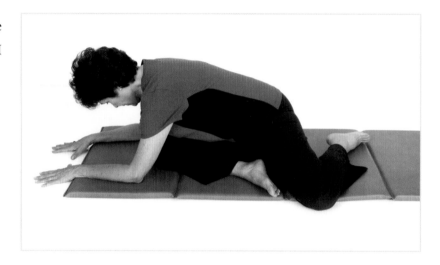

PIGEON II POSE: SINGLE-LEG PIGEON POSE

BENEFITS: *An excellent hip opener. My classes love to swoop down into this posture at the end of the day. Gives a deep, restorative stretch to the hips, seat, thighs, and chest.*

CAUTION: *If you experience any knee discomfort, direct your knee a little to the right or left or sit on a higher pillow.*

- After you have gone through the steps of Pigeon I Pose, continue to slide your right knee forward between your hands, and lower your right hip to floor. Slip a folded blanket under your right hip, if needed.

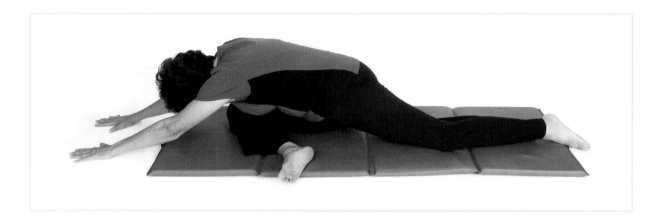

- Extend your left leg straight back behind you. Look at your back leg, making sure your leg and foot are straight. Slide your hands forward and lie flat over your right thigh.

- Doing the three Rs while in Pigeon II Pose can be very effective. While lying over your thigh, gently your press arms and back leg into the mat for Resistance . . . hold two or three breaths. Release . . . Relax . . . and slide arms out further in front of you . . . melt into the pose, open deeper to Restretch . . . (remember, happy knees!) . . . hold for six to eight breaths. Then walk your hands in and repeat the pose on the opposite side.

SOLO NESTING PIGEON POSE (*KAPOTASANA*)

Warm up well for this strong spinal rotation. This movement stretches many muscles, plus layers of fascia that separate the muscle layers and surround internal organs in your abdominal cavity.

Try this Solo Nesting Pigeon Pose as a progression of Pigeon Pose. It is a strong movement suitable for beginners and experienced students. It can easily be done solo or with a partner. Do this posture slowly and carefully.

USE THE FOLLOWING WARMUPS:

Shoulder Preparation for Garuda Arms
   (page 56)

Barn Door: Piriformus Stretch (page 66)

Little Mermaid Series (pages 72–73)

Torso Twist I and II (pages 153–155)

Pigeon I and II Poses (page 146)

PART ONE

- Sit in beginning Pigeon Pose, with your left knee folded about 90 degrees. Turn your chest slightly to the left and lean forward over your left thigh, supporting yourself on your left arm, bending that elbow, palm to the floor.

- Reach your right arm across your chest, with your palm facing up. Your left arm will bend more, lowering your trunk toward the floor. This position is already a dandy stretch. Without forcing, feel your natural stopping place.

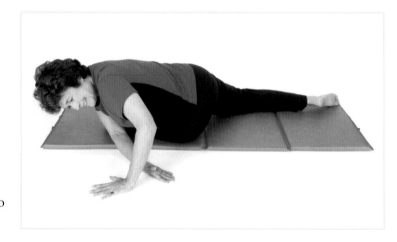

PART TWO

- Now try the three Rs. Use your torso muscles to press your supporting arm into the floor for a little Resistance for five to eight breaths. Visualize that you are pulling all the slithery organs from left to right. Pause . . . Relax . . . breathe in (a short breath, due to your restricted rib cage). Exhaling, pull the top (left) shoulder farther away from the floor. If you can, slide your right arm a little farther under yourself.

- Release. Pull your left arm out, and return both hands to the floor. Lower your chest slowly down above your left thigh. Observe. You are closer to the floor than when you began. Bravo! Repeat on the opposite side.

Downward-Facing Dog (*Adho Mukha Svanasana*)

PART ONE

USE THE FOLLOWING WARMUPS:

Table Pose with Cat and Cow (page 143)

Hamstrings Solo (page 59)

Downward-Facing Dog with a Chair (page 69)

- From Table Pose, sit back on your heels and stretch your arms straight out toward the end of the mat, spreading your fingers out like a star. Keep your hands exactly where they are, then return to Table Pose.

- From Table Pose, try to keep the curve in your lower back as you lift your knees off the mat, coming halfway into Dog. Your heels should be off the mat, and your knees soft. Yes, this step feels awkward, but stay with it. Press your hands into the mat. Your head is between your upper arms. Try bringing one heel at a time to the floor.

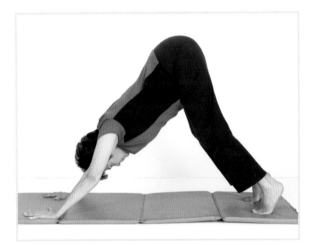

- Come out of the posture. Rest your shoulders and arms in Child's Pose.

PART TWO

- Go through the steps of part one. Be sure your weight is evenly distributed throughout your hands as you exhale, sending your hips back. Continue lengthening your spine. Lift your sit bones. Now enjoyably straighten your legs, both heels close to the mat. Breathe comfortably. Check your position. Be light on your wrists. Close the gates of your shoulders; they should be back and down, and your spine long. Hold. Enjoy for several breaths.

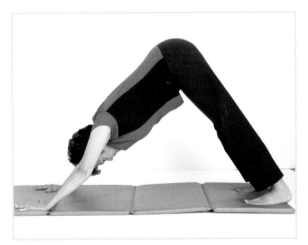

- Release and rest. Come to your knees, lower your seat toward your heels, hands to your feet, torso to thighs, forehead to floor. Enjoy this moment of relaxation. You are now resting in Child's Pose (page 164).

HALF CAMEL (*USTRASANA*)

When I first did Camel Pose, in my mid-30s, there was absolutely no way I could touch both my hands to my heels. Indeed, yoga gets better with age! Today, I pay attention to the "pieces" of Camel, warming up each piece well: arms, upper back, neck, abdomen, spine, and so on. Be creative with your choices. Take your time choosing your warmups. The joy is in the journey. Also take your time with this challenging mighty back bend. You may never need to go any further than Half Camel.

CAUTION: *If you have back problems or bone density issues, omit this posture.*

USE THE FOLLOWING WARMUPS:

Singing Snake (page 51)

Chest Expander (page 52)

Cobra Pose (pages 162–163)

Side Cobra (page 166)

Bridge with Three Rs (page 156)

Rolling Pin Series (pages 74–75)

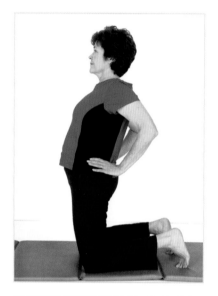

- Kneel on your mat, with your knees slightly wider than your hips. Place a folded towel beneath your knees, if needed. Turn your toes under. Place both hands on your waist, with your thumbs touching on your back. Lift up your heart. Close the gates of your shoulders, and press your hips gently forward. Involve your seat-belt muscles.

- Turn slightly to your left and lean back, grasping your left heel with your left hand. While holding on to your heel, pivot your torso so your chest faces upward. (Be sure there's no lower back discomfort.) Again, gently press your pelvis forward, elongating through your spine. Be sure you are breathing. In-hale, and raise your right arm straight out in front. Look at your thumb. Exhale.

- Inhale, and lift your right arm up to the ceiling. Continue breathing short, supportive breaths. If your lower back and shoulders still feel good . . . arch your back and look to the ceiling (do not drop your head back). Continue to breathe. Hold for two or three breaths.

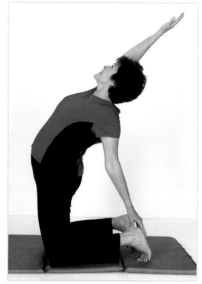

- To come out of the posture and end up in the beginning position, press your fingers into your left heel for leverage, and press your hips forward. No twisting. Repeat these steps on the opposite side.

FULL CAMEL (*USTRASANA*)

CAUTION: I have seen students faint in this Full Camel pose because they forget to breathe. So, your mantra for this and all poses is: Remember to remember to breathe!

- Begin in Half Camel Pose. Both feet and toes are turned under, your left hand holding your left heel. Are you breathing? Yes!

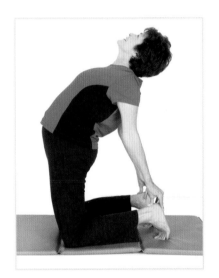

- Now reach your right hand back to grasp your right heel. Close the gates of your shoulders. Lift up your heart. Elongate your spine. Mindfully press your pubic bone forward to increase the arch. Close the blades of your shoulders.

- Very gently, look up to the ceiling. *Do not* drop your head back—that's too much stress on the neck vertebrae. Just gaze at the ceiling or a wall in front of you as you hold the posture, but do not hold your breath.

- A gentle way to release this mighty back bend is a slight turn to the left, release your right hand, then release your left hand. Sit back on your heels.

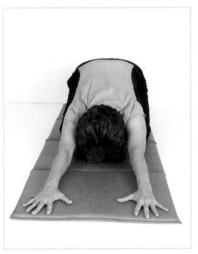

- Do Mecca Pose (page 115). Sit on your heels, stretching your arms way out or bringing them alongside your feet. This is a counter-pose; it releases and relaxes the muscles you've just used. It feels really nice to do.

- To add more heat to this pose, repeat it with your knees closer together and the tops of your feet to the mat.

THUNDERBOLT (*VAJRASANA*)

BENEFITS: *This is a nice move after deep back bends like Camel Pose. It helps bring the body back into neutral gear after a strenuous posture. As you release the pose, imagine your life current running from the base of your spine to the top of your head. In Salutation to the Moon (page 218), this pose is named Ascending Moon and can help slide you in and out of Cobra Pose (page 162), soothing the back tightness after Cobra.*

- Begin by kneeling on your mat, knees and feet hip-width apart, the tops of your feet to the mat. Sit back on your heels, using a towel on your calves for comfort if you like. Let your ankles stretch out. Hang your arms straight down at your sides.

- Inhaling, lift your hips and sweep your arms up and over your head. Keep your arms shoulder-width apart, palms facing one another. Lean slightly back and look up toward the energy between your hands. Smile.

- Exhaling, sit on your heels again, fold your chest to your thighs, and sweep your arms behind your back into Child's Pose. Repeat the two motions—lifting up, then folding back down—six to eight times. Then rest in Child's Pose for 1 minute.

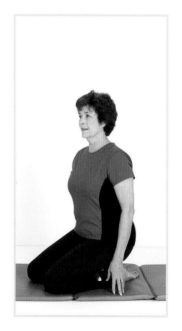
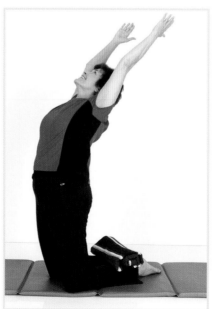
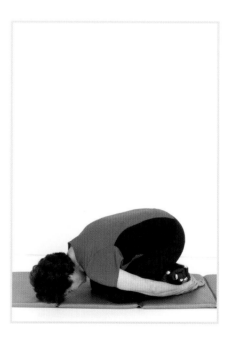

TORSO TWIST I (*PARIVARTANASANA*)

BENEFITS: *This posture lets you "wring out" your liver, kidneys, and intestines like a washcloth.*

CAUTION: *Approach all twists with caution if you suffer from disc problems anywhere in your spine.*

YIN TIP: *This first little move is important. It helps the spine remain straight and aligned (not arched back) for the final position.*

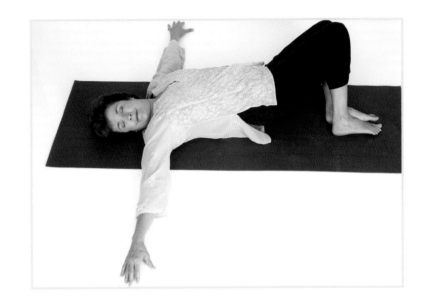

- Begin by lying on your mat, with your knees bent and feet on the mat. Lift your hips ¼ inch off mat, swish them 2 inches or so to the right, then place your hips back on the mat. Your spine will remain at this angle throughout the posture. Extend your arms into a T, palms turned down.

- Exhaling, slowly lower your bent legs to the left, while your head turns right. Place a pillow between or beneath your knees for more comfort.

- Repeat three times, then on the last twist, *hold* for six to eight breaths. Enjoy the feeling of the pose. Breathe energy slowly in, and send it to the ends of your toes and fingers on the exhale.

- Return to the beginning, and swish your hips to the left. Follow the above steps with both knees falling to the right, and look over your left shoulder. Repeat three times and *hold* the last twist six to eight breaths.

- Return to center. Close your eyes, and scan your body. Enjoy the sensations of this posture.

TORSO TWIST II (*JATHARA PARIVRITTI*)

BENEFITS: *Tones abdominal organs, stretches and lengthens connecting tissue and muscles across the belly, and tones back and hips. Has an immediate calming effect on nervous system. Both Torso Twist I and Torso Twist II can be used as fabulous yin warmups for all twisting poses.*

USE THE FOLLOWING WARMUPS:

Torso Twist I and II (pages 153–155)

Ring the Gong (page 55)

YIN TIP: *Remind yourself: This posture is not about how far I can push my knee to the floor. Keep your witness close by.*

CAUTION: *Placing your spine at a slight angle, as in the first step, ensures that it will remain straight and long in the final position. Not angling the spine first can cause overarching and pain in the final step.*

- Begin by lying on your back with your knees bent, feet on the mat, and spine center. Extend your arms to form a T, palms up. Lift your hips ¼ inch off the mat, swish your hips to the right about 2 inches, and return your hips to the mat. Your spine is now on an angle.

- Slowly straighten your right leg. Using your right hand, pull your left knee toward your right armpit, lifting your foot off the mat. Relax your shoulders. Hold for two or three breaths.

- Push your thigh away from your chest a few inches. Place your right hand outside of your left thigh. Slowly drop your bent knee across your body. Guide your knee to its natural stopping point. Hold. Observe the distance between your knee and the floor. No forcing. No bouncing. Just witness. Your shoulder stays on the mat. Look over left shoulder.

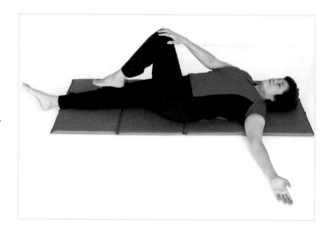

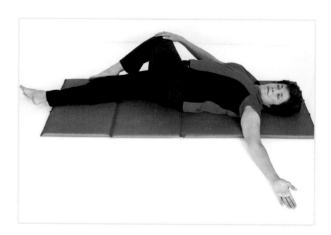

YIN TIP: *If you're stiff, rest your bent knee on a cushion. As you progress (and you will!), reduce its thickness.*

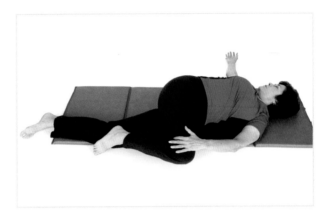

- Now add the three Rs. This is where it gets interesting! All the three Rs are done with tuning in to your witness self. Truly listen to your body each step of the way. One-pointed attention is here as well. Holding on to your bent leg with one hand, gently press it *away* from you, against the Resistance of your hand for three or four breaths. The leg does not move. Imagine . . . *feel* . . . the Saran Wrap abdominal fascia moving from left to right. Hold for five breaths. Relax . . . breathe in. Exhaling, Re-stretch. You guide your knee, no pushing, into its new natural stopping place.

- To get more out of the last step, still holding the outside of your bent leg, very gently push the leg toward your hand. Be conscious of using back and waist muscles, *not* your hip muscle, to press back. Relax . . . breathe in. Exhaling slowly, guide your bent leg effortlessly closer to the floor. Your limit is when your opposite shoulder lifts off the mat. Hold for three or four breaths. Return your spine to the center of the mat. Now go through these steps on the opposite side.

BRIDGE POSE (*Setu Bandha*)

BENEFITS: *Frequently prescribed by health care practitioners as part of back-strengthening programs. Will improve your posture and breathing. Extremely effective when done slowly, emphasizing breath rather than repeated mechanically. Definitely a core Desert Island posture for students over 50, it prepares you for back bends like Camel Pose (pages 150–151) and inverted postures like Half Shoulderstand (pages 193–194).*

- Lie on your back, with your knees bent (no discomfort), feet hip-width apart, heels comfortably close to your seat, your hands down alongside your body. Rest in this posture; watch your breathing. Take a few complete breaths.

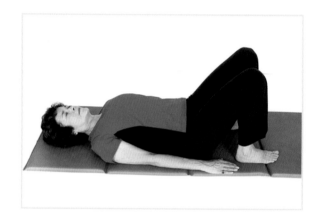

- Again, slowly, enjoyably, inhale . . . feel your ribs expand . . . then on the exhale . . . press your feet into the mat. Feel your lower back pleasantly lengthen . . . continue drawing your tailbone under . . . until your seat muscle naturally begins to lift off the mat.

- Feet are in line with hips . . . press down into your feet and slowly peel your spine off the mat, one vertebra at a time.

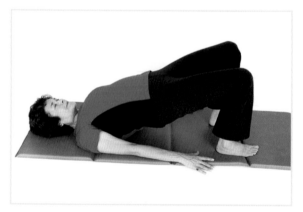

- Continue pressing into your feet . . . remain comfortably in the pose. Close the gates of the shoulders. Breathe in a little deeper . . . feel your back, seat, and thigh muscles softly contracting, strengthening. Exhaling, release your spine slowly back down to the mat. Repeat two or three times.

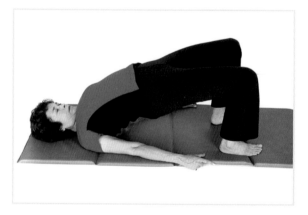

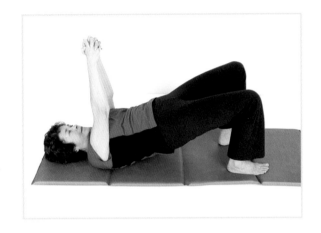

● Variation: In the first step, instead of your hands resting on the floor, raise both arms up to the ceiling and clasp your hands above your chest. Hold your arms in this position while you complete the remainder of the pose. Once you've lowered your spine back down, slowly lower your arms. Wonderful for releasing tension between your shoulder blades.

CAUTION: *In the final step, lower your hips if you feel back discomfort. There is no pain whatsoever in this pose!*

YIN TIP: *To improve your Bridge Pose, use the three Rs as you go through the steps. In the final step, Resist, firmly pressing your shoulders, arms, and hands and feet into the mat. Contract your thighs and abdomen; tighten facial muscles. Hold for two or three breaths. It takes concentration (dharana) and nonviolence (ahimsa) to be sure Resistance is without strain and even throughout your whole body. Relax, breathe in . . . Now Restretch . . . go a little higher . . . lift off heels, close the gates of the shoulders . . . breathe deeply in . . . feel your chest open like a flower . . . enjoy . . . hold for two or three breaths, then release. Come out of pose . . . one vertebra at a time. Bring both knees to chest, rock from side to side for about 30 seconds. Stop, place your feet to the floor, and rest.*

HAPPY BABY POSE WITH THREE RS (*SUPTA EKAPADASANA*)

- Lie faceup, with your knees bent and feet to the mat. Raise your right leg and, if you wish, place a belt or your right hand around the outer edge of your foot (you may also put your left hand on the back of your right thigh). Bend your right knee 90 degrees. Place a pillow beneath your head, if needed. Close your eyes and hold this enjoyable stretch for two or three breaths.

USE THE FOLLOWING WARMUPS:

Knee to Chest with Three Rs (page 64)

Dancing the Star (page 113)

Barn Door: Piriformus Stretch (page 66)

Frog Pose (page 115)

- Now apply the three Rs. Gently but steadily push your right foot up into your right hand or the belt. At the same time, pull your right hand or belt downward to create resistance. Hold the Resistance, no bouncing, for six breaths. Relax. Feel the relaxation happening. Now Restretch . . . take your time. Guide your own thigh or knee toward your right armpit and ribs. Keep your lower back to mat. For those who are flexible, your foot could go back over your head. Hold for three to six breaths. Happy Baby is worth practicing. It always makes me smile. Repeat on the opposite leg.

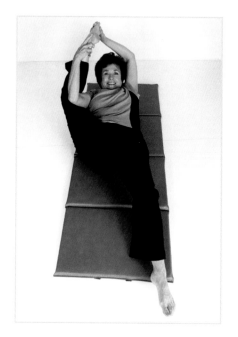

- Variation: Raise your right leg, and instead of holding the foot with the right hand, grab on to your toes with the left (opposite) hand. Place your right elbow in the crook of your knee, your forearm along your calf, your right hand holding on to the back of your ankle. Lift your head off the mat and gently pull your leg toward your head.

- Variation: Straighten your left leg as you work with the right.

REALLY HAPPY BABY (*SUPTA EKAPADASANA*)

Changing my grandchildren's diapers has made me appreciate how this posture captures the innocence, flexibility, and wonder of being a happy baby.

CAUTION: *Not a pose to be done with disc problems.*

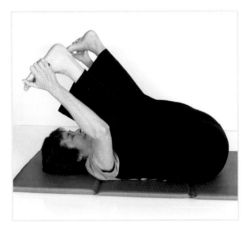

- After you have done each leg separately in Happy Baby, do both legs. Lie faceup and raise both legs, bending the knees 90 degrees. Use belts or your hands to grasp the outer edges of your feet. Press your knee toward your open armpits, keeping your lower back and hips on the mat. Hold the pose, breathing comfortably.

Anchored Boat Pose (*Ardha Navasana*)

Benefits: *Strengthens core abdominals. A safe challenge. Stimulates internal organs.*

Caution: *If you have lower back problems, be cautious. Remember to buckle your seat belt. To avoid back strain, lift one leg at a time in the second step, keeping the other foot on the floor.*

- Sit tall with your knees bent and feet on the mat. Lean back onto your elbows. Chest is open. You can spread your fingers wide for added support. Anchor your abs by pulling in your core muscles behind your navel. Keep them anchored, as they support your back.

- Keeping your knees bent, lift your legs (one at a time, if your lower back needs help) and bring your shins parallel to the floor. Look at your toes. They should be in line with your knees. Smile at them, and hold for three to six breaths with no strain and no pain.

- Release the pose, and return to the beginning. Relax. Inhaling, arch your spine, open the chest, lift up your heart, and look up. Take a deep, wonderful breath in. Release, and repeat all the steps.

- Variation: Before releasing the pose, extend your legs all the way up toward the ceiling. Your feet are relaxed, not pointed or flexed. Continue to breathe. Smile at your toes. Relax your shoulders as you hold for three breaths or longer. Work toward holding the pose comfortably for longer and longer periods of time.

- Variation: Anchored Boat position can easily be turned into another creative way to strengthen the abs. For more ab heat, try bicycling with your legs while in this pose, 10 times each leg.

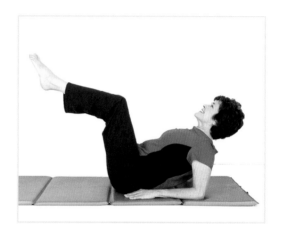

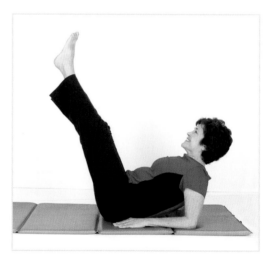

SPHINX POSE

BENEFITS: *Increases flexibility and strength in the arms, chest, and shoulders. Emphasizes opening the front chest, assisting muscles for breathing, and good posture. Stimulates kidneys and adrenals.*

CAUTION: *Lower-back problems? Separate your legs wider than your hips, heels turned out.*

USE THE FOLLOWING WARMUPS:

Rolling Pin Series (pages 74–75)

Chest Expander (page 52)

Cat and Cow Pose (page 114)

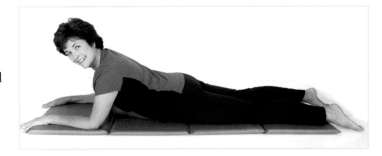

- Lie on your abdomen, with your feet hip-width apart and the tops of your feet on the mat. Bend your elbows and place your forearms on the mat. Slide your elbows beneath your armpits, palms down, and spread your fingers.

- Press your forearms into the mat, and lift your collarbone. Exhaling, slowly turn your head to the right . . . pause . . . return to center. Exhaling, turn your head to the left . . . pause . . . return to center. Now, slowly drop your head forward . . . hold for two or three breaths . . . Exhale, lower your torso back to the mat . . . rest for two or three breaths.

Cobra Pose (*Bhujangasana*)

Benefits: *Breaks up tension in the back and shoulders. Increases strength and flexibility of spine and arms. Stimulates kidneys and adrenals.*

Caution: *No pain in these postures. Moving the hands farther forward makes Cobra less difficult. Seat muscles can be either firm or soft, whatever feels best for you and your back.*

USE THE FOLLOWING WARMUPS

Rolling Pin Series (pages 74–75)

Chest Expander (page 52)

Thunderbolt (page 152)

Mecca Pose (page 115)

Sphinx Pose (page 161)

Cat and Cow Pose (page 114)

LOW COBRA POSE

- Lie on your abdomen with your legs hip-width apart, tops of your feet to the mat. Place arms as in Sphinx Pose, with elbows beneath armpits. Now place your palms on the mat where your elbows were. Elbows are now bent, close to your body.

- Place your forehead to the mat, and roll your shoulders back and down. Close gates of shoulders.

- Inhaling, lengthen your neck and engage the back muscles. Be sure weight is even throughout your hands, and press your palms into the floor . . . slowly raising your chest and head. Your gaze is straight ahead.

- Open the eyes of the heart . . . shoulders back and down . . . seat muscle active, not tight. In Low Cobra, you keep the top of your pelvis to the mat, elbows slightly bent. This will keep pressure out of lower back. Hold for one breath. Repeat at least three to five times, inhaling slowly up and exhaling down.

- The three Rs will prepare the body for Full Cobra and Locust poses. It is achieved by first resting on Sphinx elbows. Rock your body from side to side, five or six times; no tension, just enjoy. This helps side muscles to relax. Now pause . . . begin to Resist . . . press your forearms steadily into the mat . . . press tops of feet (gently) downward, tightening legs. Use resistance to contract chest, shoulders, arms, back, and seat muscles. Hold for three to five breaths. Let a little Sphinx smile come to your lips . . . now Relax . . . feel muscles go limp . . . Restretch . . . Repeat the steps of Low Cobra again. Observe any differences in ease and fluidity of pose.

Yin Tip: *Making Cobra Pose more comfortable does not make it less powerful. Try placing a firm pillow or folded blanket underneath your rib cage and hips. Slide the blanket edge about 6 inches above your navel. All of the Cobra preparations lead you into Locust Pose.*

FULL COBRA POSE

CAUTION: *Too often I see students of all ages tolerate pain in this pose. Everybody is different. Please, omit Full Cobra and stay in pain-free Low Cobra.*

- Palms to mat . . . thumbs near armpits . . . forehead to mat. Go through your checklist: shoulders back and down, shoulder gates closed, neck long, weight even throughout hands, light contraction in seat muscles.

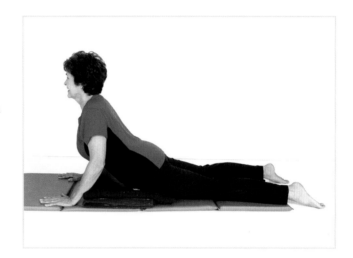

- Inhale, engage your back muscles, press palms, raise chest and head away from mat . . . shoulders back and down. Now curve deeper into the pose. Elbows stay bent . . . use arms for balance and for engaging your deep back muscles for strength. Your navel will be off the mat.

- Move slowly up and down, coordinating movement with your breathing, at least five times. Then try holding Cobra Pose for three or four breaths. Back of your neck is long . . . gaze to the floor. The three Rs you did for Low Cobra should really help this pose feel fluid and comfortable as you hold the final step.

- Exhaling, come out of Cobra slowly . . . no rush . . . turn your head to the side. Go into Child's Pose (page 164). Enjoy the sensations of Cobra Pose as you rest.

CHILD'S POSE (*BALASANA*) WITH RING THE GONG

Also called Mecca Pose or Folded Leaf, this is a resting posture, also called a counter-pose, which means stretching in the opposite direction—for example, after back bends such as Cobra and Camel poses. Tapping Muscles or Ring the Gong releases muscle tightness and feels good.

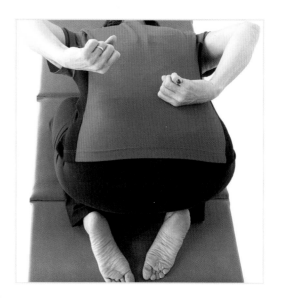

- Sit on your heels, and lay your torso over your thighs, forehead to floor. Open your thighs so you can breathe comfortably . . . hands touch ankles. This is Child's Pose.

- Now, Ring the Gong . . . hands in two gentle fists, reach up and tap the lower back muscles. Tap . . . tap . . . tap . . . for three or four breaths.

LOCUST POSE (SHALABHASANA)

BENEFITS: *Strengthens entire torso as well as lower-back, seat, and leg muscles. Improves digestion and elimination.*

USE THE FOLLOWING WARMUPS:

Stargazing Yogoda (page 111)

Sphinx Pose with Three Rs (page 161)

YIN TIP: *Making Locust Pose more comfortable does not make it less powerful. Try placing a firm pillow or folded blanket underneath your rib cage and hips. Place the blanket edge about 2 inches below your navel, with your chest on the mat. All of the Cobra preparations lead you into Locust.*

CAUTION: *This pose is challenging. If you feel back or neck pain, do not lift your leg so high or completely omit this posture. Remember—no pain.*

- Lie on your abdomen with your legs hip-width apart and tops of feet to the floor. Rest your forehead or cheek to the mat. Extend your arms alongside your torso, palms down, or fold them under your forehead.

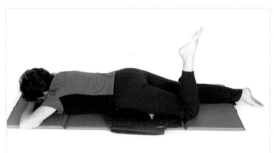

- Bend your left knee. Foot is relaxed, toes gently pointing to ceiling.

- Exhaling, lift your left knee off the mat, pause . . . inhale, lower knee to floor. Repeat three times each leg.

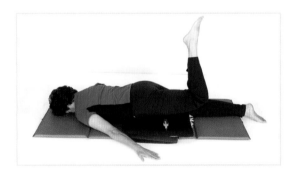

- Repeat the above steps, then, exhaling, raise your left leg with your knee bent, pause . . . now slowly straighten your left leg. Hold for two or three breaths, and lower your leg. Then repeat all the steps on the right leg.

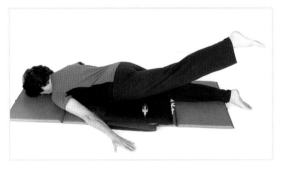

- Now do both legs. Exhaling, raise both knees up, then straighten the legs. Hold for two or three breaths.

SIDE COBRA (*BHUJANGASANA*)

USE THE FOLLOWING WARMUPS:

Spider on the Wall (pages 204–205)

Chest Expander (page 52)

Rolling Pin Series (pages 74–75)

- Begin in Cobra Pose (page 162). Roll over onto your left side. Extend your left arm out, hand below the line of the shoulder, palm to floor. Be sure your shoulders and your left breast are comfortable.

- Arch your spine and press your chest forward, pulling the right (top) arm back, arms forming a V, palms to ceiling. Open your chest, close the gates of the shoulders. Enjoy! Hold for two or three breaths. Support your head with a block, if needed. Repeat on the opposite side.

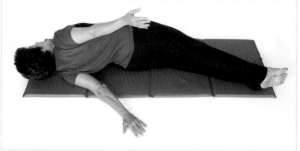

SIDE BOW POSE (*DHANURASANA*)

YIN TIP: *If you are straining, wait a few months and try again. Give your muscles and connecting tissues a chance to stretch out.*

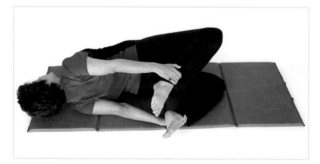

- Add a little heat to your Side Cobra Pose. While on your left side, hold your left ankle with your left hand, and hold your right ankle with your right hand. Hold for 15 to 30 seconds on each side.

- Then, roll in Side Bow from side to side. Release, and go into Seed Pose (opposite page), then Mecca Pose (page 115), followed by Seated Forward Bend (page 172). Rest.

SEED POSE

A relaxation pose, usually done on the right side so as not to squeeze the heart, is comfortable. Seed is also a transition posture—it helps you go smoothly from lying down to sitting up. Look for the deeper meaning within Seed Pose. Take a moment to ponder the essence, the powerful life force within every little seed. Ponder for a moment the essence, the powerful life force within you.

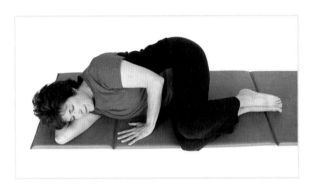

- Lie on your right side . . . make a pillow out of your right arm. Bring your knees into your chest. Rest for three or four breaths.

- To sit up, place your left hand on the floor in front of your chest. Lean forward, and use your arms to press yourself up. Head (your thinking) is the last to come up.

CHATARANGA I

BENEFITS: *Strengthens both front and back of body. A safe, challenging posture. Sends a message to all the bones of your body to remain strong and retain calcium. You'll be surprised, when you fit all the pieces of this pose together, how easy it is to do.*

USE THE FOLLOWING WARMUPS:

Spider on the Wall (pages 204–205)

Downward-Facing Dog (page 149)

Cobra Pose (pages 162–163)

Flying Sunbird (page 144)

Stargazing Situp (page 48)

Sphinx Pose (page 161)

Anchored Boat Pose (page 160)

● Begin in Sphinx Pose (page 161), on your abdomen, feet hip-width apart, toes turned under so you are *not* on the tops of your feet. Bend your elbows, bringing your forearms to the mat. Spread your fingers to form a star. Roll the weight evenly toward the center of your hand and arm bones.

● Pull your seat-belt muscles inward. Breathe in and, exhaling, press down on your forearms and lift *only* your hips off the mat. Hold, with shallow breathing for four to six breaths. Relax. Rest for a moment. Continue.

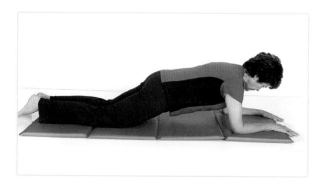

● Repeat the last step, but this time, with active legs and seat. Pull your kneecaps up and contract your thigh muscles (legs will be slightly off mat). Exhaling, press down on your forearms and hands (for elbow comfort, roll arm bones inward). Core abdominals help you lift hips and legs off the mat. Use your toes. Your body now forms a line as straight as a stick. Be sure your core abdominals are supporting you—that is, don't point your seat up to the ceiling, and don't sway your belly to the floor. Hold for a few breaths, or 30 seconds, gazing at the floor.

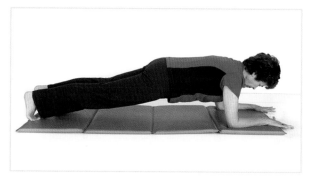

● Release and relax. Turn onto your right side, knees to chest; right arm pillows your head in Seed Pose. Close your eyes. Feel Chataranga I still vibrating through your body.

SAGE TWIST (*MARICHYASANA*)

BENEFITS: *Our internal organs love to be squeezed. Like water being squeezed from a washcloth, while in a twist, you pulse circulation throughout your internal organs and connecting tissue.*

USE THE FOLLOWING WARMUPS:

Salutation to the Hips (page 216)

Torso Twist I and II (pages 153–155)

YIN TIP: *Sage Twist can be done in a chair or in your car. Changing the leg position makes the twist a little more difficult.*

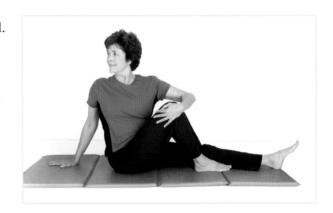

- Sit on the mat, with both legs extended forward. Bend your right knee and place your right foot on the mat just to the inside of your left thigh, toes pointing forward. To make this pose more difficult, place your right foot to the *outside* of your left thigh. Place your right hand behind you for balance. Wrap your left palm around the outside of your right knee. Inhale . . . extend . . . lift your spine upward.

- Exhaling . . . spiral your torso to the right . . . then, turn your head right. Stop here.

YIN TIP: *Slowly and gently turn your head right and left a few times. Observe this move—it has nothing to do with turning your torso.*

- Clasp your right hand over your left. The three Rs can be used with ease here. Remember the three elements: first contract your hip and abdomen gently, then hold the Resistance for six breaths, steady, no bouncing. Press it away from you (Resist). Your hands will form a little wall to push against. Pause . . . Relax . . . breathe in . . . exhale, relaxing the muscles involved. Lift your spine upwards, then Restretch a little further . . . sitting tall . . . feel how much further you can spiral into a safe twist.

HERO'S TWIST (*VIRASANA*)

Hero's Twist is a little different from other twists, as you'll soon experience. The warmups are an important preparation for this fun twist. The three Rs are a great addition for getting the most from this posture.

BENEFITS: *A challenging, deep stretch for hips. Leads you directly into stillness.*

YIN TIP: *Sit on a cushion if both sit bones do not contact the floor.*

USE THE FOLLOWING WARMUPS:

Barn Door: Piriformus Stretch (page 66)

Salutation to the Hips (page 216)

Torso Twist I and II (pages 153–155)

Pigeon I Pose (page 146)

Little Mermaid Series (pages 72–73)

Sage Twist (page 169)

- Sit tall. Bring your left thigh over your right bent knee. Both sit bones and outsides of feet are to the floor. Turn your chest toward the right, lean forward over your left thigh. (Note photo.) Place your hands to the floor. Enjoy the hips stretching. Hold for three or four breaths.

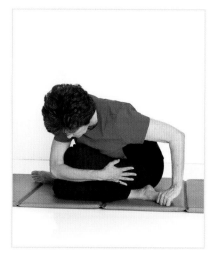

- Wrap your right forearm around your left knee. Feel your thigh touch your ribs. Hold on to your thigh with both arms, and hug it to your chest as you slowly sit up. Clasping the knee as close to your chest as possible, keep your spine long, and slowly sit up straight and tall. Feel this strong stretch in your hip.

- Now do the three Rs. Resist. Gently press your left knee into your right forearm. Hold steady for three or four breaths. Relax . . . breathe in. Again . . . Resist . . . Exhale. Pull your soft internal
organs from the right to the left. Hold for two or three breaths . . . Relax . . . Breathe in . . . Now, Restretch . . . Lengthen and lift your spine. Exhale . . . go a little deeper into Hero's Twist. Hold for two or three breaths. Notice how far you've gone.

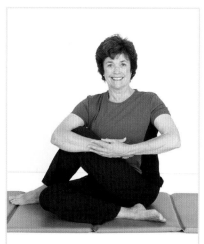

- Release. Sit with your ankles crossed. Close your eyes. Observe sensations within your body. Repeat on the opposite side. Note which side is tighter. Next time you practice, begin with the tighter side. Soon both sides will be of similar flexibility.

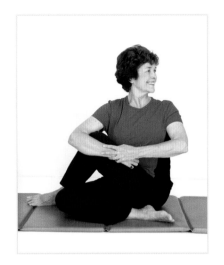

- To deepen the hip and abdominal stretch, repeat the steps above. While doing the three Rs, press your left leg gently away from your chest, holding the leg without letting it move for two or three breaths. Relax . . . stop, breathe in, relaxing the muscles involved. Restretch, go into Hero's Twist a little deeper, lifting up the spine, spiraling further on the exhale. Imagine the sheath of fascia stretching from right to left . . . look over your left shoulder . . . hold for two or three more breaths.
Relax . . . return to center. Undo your legs . . . sit with your ankles crossed. Close your eyes. Dive into the stillness. Enjoy it . . . for 1 minute. When you are ready, repeat on the opposite side.

SEATED FORWARD BEND (*PASCHIMOTTANASANA*)

BENEFITS: *Like a flower that closes in the evening to rest, this posture has a calming, quieting effect on body and mind. Seated Forward Bend internally stretches the entire back of the body, and tones and increases circulation to abdominal organs.*

This classic yoga pose is made up of many pieces. Like a puzzle, when one piece is too tight, the effect detracts from the whole picture. Common tight areas are hips, lower back, hamstrings, calf muscles, and the soles of your feet. Doing the warmups first will significantly improve this (and any) yoga posture. Courage! Every midlife body is stiff when beginning forward bends. It feels good to move into the posture, then hold the pose.

USE THE FOLLOWING WARMUPS:

Hamstrings Solo (page 59)

Hamstrings 3-Ways (page 59)

Barn Door: Piriformus Stretch (page 66)

Wall Calf Stretch (page 65)

Salutation to the Hips (page 216)

Striding Forward Bend (page 178)

Fun with Fascia (page 35)

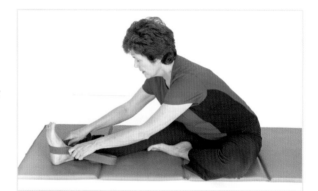

- Sit on your mat with your legs extended comfortably in front of you. Now bend your left knee, placing your left foot against your right inner thigh. Reach down with your hands and pull your seat muscles backward so that you are sitting directly on your sit bones. Sit tall. Lift up your heart.

- Inhaling, raise both arms up; fingers point to ceiling. Soften your right leg.

- Exhaling, fold forward from the hip hinge. Aim your chest, hands, and head toward your right foot.

YIN TIP: *You may also use a yoga belt wrapped around your foot, as in the photo, to help your stretch.*

- Hands can touch thigh, knee, ankle, or foot. To release your back, slide your hands beneath your knee, palms down, and bend your knee a little.

- Now, repeat the steps. Go back and forth, in rhythm with your breath, three times. Stop . . . hold in the final step for six to eight breaths. Then repeat with the other leg.

REVOLVING HEAD TO KNEE (*PARIVRTTA JANU SIRSASANA*)

BENEFITS: *Increased circulation to internal organs. Nice stretch for hamstrings and back.*

USE THE FOLLOWING WARMUPS:

Fan Pose (page 176)

Hamstrings Solo (page 59)

Hamstrings 3-Ways (page 59)

Partner Hamstring Stretch (page 198)

Triangle Pose (page 181)

Torso Twist I and II (pages 153–155)

Seated Forward Bend (opposite page)

● While sitting on the mat, begin by extending your right leg straight out in front . . . bend your left knee, placing the left foot comfortably on (or away from) your right inner thigh. Lift up your arms, lift up your heart, and with a long back, fold forward over your extended leg, finding your outstretched foot with your hands. Hold for four to eight breaths.

YIN TIP: *Don't be discouraged if you cannot reach your foot without rounding your shoulders and back. Loop a belt or towel around your foot, if needed, using the steady leverage of the belt. Partner Seated Side Bend helps this posture dramatically.*

● Now become more revolved by going into a simple twist. Sit tall (Janu Sirsana), turn your torso toward your bent left knee, placing right hand on bent left knee, left hand to floor. Exhale into an easy twist. Spiraling in the opposite direction before going into Sirsasana makes it easier.

● Now, leaning right, place your right arm inside your right thigh, elbow down, palm facing up. Reach up with your left arm; bring it close to your ear.

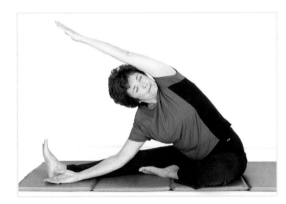

● If your elbow will not reach the floor, use a bolster or block under your elbow to help open the chest, or hold on to a belt looped around your right foot. Imagine all inner the organs moving, pulling, squeezing from right to left . . . hold for six to eight breaths. The three Rs work beautifully in this step. Resist, and push left ribs gently up. Holding on to a belt or your leg helps the resistance. Hold for three breaths. Relax. Breath in, Restretch . . . and with ease, extend over your right leg. Repeat on the opposite side.

SACRED MOUNTAIN POSE (*TADASANA*)

Sacred Mountain Pose is the foundation of all standing poses. It acknowledges new beginnings, the present moment, and is therefore considered sacred.

Read the directions over slowly. I realize that for a simple posture, the directions are long. Take one or two details you enjoy and use them that day, then vary the details. Make your own interpretations and insights. Keep this posture fresh and interesting.

Tadasana is returning home. Home is the place within you of both heart and hearth. Tadasana is a transition pose—it helps you make the transition from the parking lot, your efforts to make class on time, then move from posture to posture to posture, returning again and again to the sacred moment of now.

Let this posture help you settle into your body, into your heart and into your inner teacher. Observe, in a flash, what you have brought with you this moment. Ask yourself, "Where am I?" Encourage your Self to welcome, rather than run, from the answers. Go out into nature and do Sacred Mountain Pose . . . feel a part of everything—earth, trees, the wind, the birds—and everything is a part of you.

Because this pose is so simple, it is easy to miss or take for granted. A Type A personality wants to say, "Let's get going! Let's do Sun Sal now!" Or, "This really isn't a posture." It takes maturing and understanding to realize . . . Sacred Mountain Pose is an important moment.

And now we begin . . .

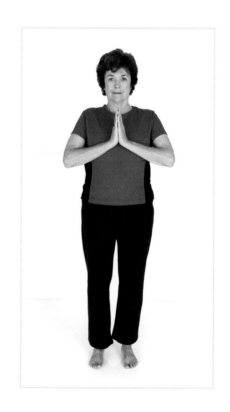

- Stand tall. Put the palms of your hands together. Eyes soft. Awaken your witness. Feel your feet to the earth. Lift your toes, then place them lightly to earth. Big toes can be touching, or your feet can be hip-width apart. Imagine your long toes growing into vines or roots . . . rooting your feet deeply into the earth. Kneecaps pulled up but not locked.

- Move your awareness up into your pelvis. Gently point your tailbone downward and pull the core muscles behind your navel back into and up your spine. These two moves are done as one, and I call them "buckling up your seat belt," because a seat belt supports and holds you safely in place. The curves of your spine are natural and flowing. Bring awareness to your shoulders. Pull them down and back from your ears, and slide your shoulder blades down as well. Lift up your heart. Create space in your chest. Your head floats lightly like a balloon above your shoulders.

- With your palms together in Namaste, nestle the knuckles of your thumbs into the little indentation in your breastbone (sternum) called the "lake of tranquillity." Bowing the head quiets the mind. Take a moment to give thanks to all the teachers in your life who have brought you to this moment in time. Feel the stirring of gratitude within the portable altar you carry in the center of your chest.

- Remain in Tadasana for six to eight breaths.

FAN POSE (*PRASARITA PADOTTANASANA*)

BENEFITS: *Fan Pose is a great warmup and also a transition posture, helping you move from one pose to another.*

- Begin in Five-Pointed Star (page 188), feet well apart and pointing forward. Extend your arms to a T or a V. Your body looks like a five-pointed star. Fold forward, extending your arms and placing your hands on the floor or blocks way out in front of you. Enjoy this stretch! At first, soften your knees. After a few weeks working with Fan Pose and other hamstring stretches, begin to engage your kneecaps and thighs.

- Now, hold on to your ankles. You are now in Fan Pose. Hold for three to six breaths.

- Variation: A lovely way to rest your back in Fan Pose is to cross your elbows and hold on to the outer thighs. Hold for 10 seconds, then cross your elbows again, holding on to outer thighs. Hold for three to six breaths.

- Walk your hands up your thighs, and return to Five-Pointed Star.

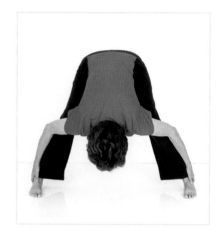

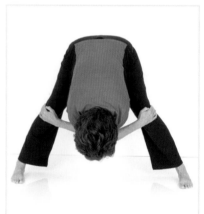

STANDING FORWARD BEND (*UTTANASANA*)

BENEFITS: *Lengthens the entire back of the body and makes space between the vertebrae of your upper neck. Gravity helps free the cervical spine and allows neck muscles to relax. Improves overall circulation and has a calming effect on body and mind.*

USE THE FOLLOWING WARMUP:

Standing Forward Bend with Block, Alternating Legs (page 61)

CAUTION: *Be very careful of all forward bends if you have unmedicated high blood pressure or disc problems. If you have any questions, check with your doctor or health professional.*

- Stand in Sacred Mountain Pose. Inhaling . . . raise your arms forward, then up overhead.

- As you exhale, sweep your arms out to the sides and bend forward from the hinge of your hips. When you feel the pull on the back of your legs, soften your knees. Let your arms hang and touch the earth ("earth" could be a block or chair in front of you). Ease your knees just a little more to relax your low back.

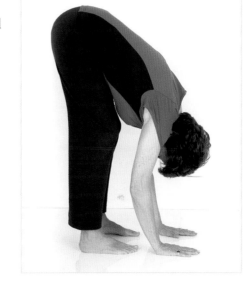

- As you inhale . . . roll up slowly . . . buckle seat belt for support . . . and then raise arms overhead.

- Repeat three more times, then stay in folded position. Pull up your kneecaps. Engage your thighs. Lift your sit bones. No bouncing! No strain!

- To come up, place your hands on your legs and "walk" them up very, very slowly. Be sure you continue to breathe. Stand tall.

YIN TIP: *If leg and back tightness make this position really uncomfortable, practice with elbows or hands on a chair seat or other support.*

STRIDING FORWARD BEND

Another favorite Desert Island posture, this is a standing, asymmetrical forward bend, meaning muscles on the right and left side of the back and hamstrings are stretched separately.

BENEFITS: *Improves balance, opens hips, stretches hamstrings, tones abdominals, releases neck tension, increases circulation to upper torso and head.*

USE THE FOLLOWING WARMUPS:

An excellent warmup on its own. Move up and down three times each side.

Hamstring stretches, done lying down or standing (page 59)

Hug a Tree (page 68)

- Stand in Sacred Mountain Pose. Exhale, and stride your left foot forward about 3 to 3½ feet. Turn your right foot slightly outward for stability. Place your hands where your upper thigh and hip bones meet. This is your hip "hinge." Now turn your hips so they are square over your right leg.

- Exhaling, fold over your hip hinge, release your hands, and let your arms hang. Enjoy this pose! If your head is not close to your right knee, bend your knee more. If you are flexible, straighten it.

- Inhale as you roll up slowly and consciously. Extend arms out to the sides, bend elbows, buckle seat belt muscles to support your rounded midback . . . use your thighs . . . and then raise arms overhead, arms near your ears. To come up safely, place your hands on your thighs and, with a rounded back, walk them up your legs.

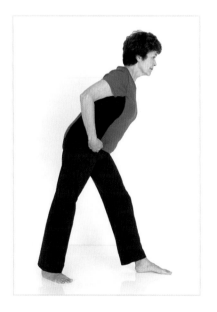
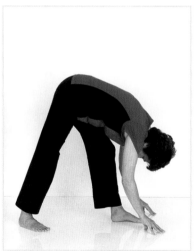
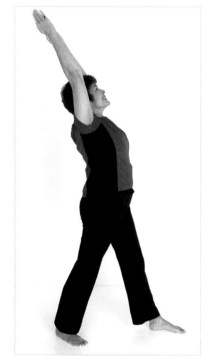

- Repeat these steps three times. Then stay in the final step for six to eight breaths. Repeat with your right foot forward.

- After a few weeks, try different arm positions. Sweep your arms out from the sides, like eagle wings, or even place them behind your low back, like a speed skater. Lower your chest toward your forward thigh, then inhale and raise your upper back until you are all the way up, lifting arms overhead.

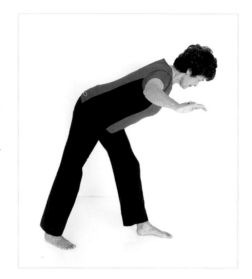

CRESCENT MOON (*ARDHA CHANDRASANA* I)

BENEFITS: *Prepares the body for Half Moon Balance (page 188).*

- Stand in Sacred Mountain Pose. Bring your feet together, ankles and big toes touching or just a few inches apart. Feel your feet rooted in the earth. Inhaling, raise your hands up to the ceiling.

- Exhaling, press your left hip and slide your rib cage to the left, and lean your body right into a Crescent Moon. As you move right, press your left foot into the mat. Relax your shoulders.

- Come back to center and repeat the steps three times on each side.

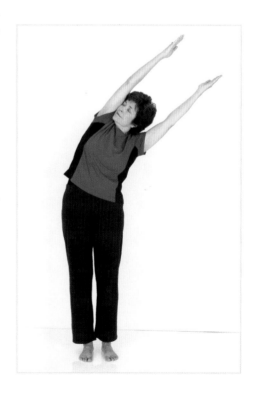

HALF CHAIR POSE

BENEFITS: *Strengthens legs, back, shoulders, and arms. Builds stamina.*

CAUTION: *If you have problem knees, you might want to skip this one. Return to it after thigh muscles get stronger.*

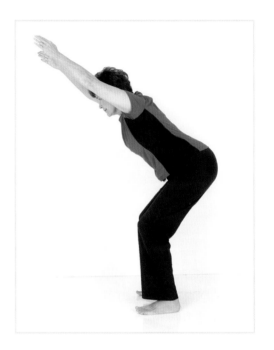

- Start in Sacred Mountain Pose. Inhaling, raise your arms forward and up and overhead, palms facing each other.

- Exhaling, bend your knees and squat halfway to the floor. As you hold for two or three breaths, remember it's important to use core abdominals like a seat belt holding you securely in your pose. So buckle up . . . pull 'em in . . . soften your arms as you keep them raised. Gaze is straight ahead. Breath is shallow.

- Repeat these steps three times. Now, hold the final step . . . for six to eight breaths.

- Remember to use your thighs, abdominals, and seat muscles to lift you up to standing, not your lower back.

TRIANGLE POSE (*UTTHITA TRIKONASANA*)

BENEFITS: *Stretches the back and backs of legs, and lengthens deep tissue connections in hips. Stretches breathing muscles between ribs, thus improving breathing capacity.*

YIN TIP: *Take a few minutes to do the warmups. They will make Triangle Pose so much more comfortable.*

USE THE FOLLOWING WARMUPS:

Victory Goddess (page 77)

Partner Seated Side Bend (page 207)

Hug a Tree (page 68)

Sage Twist (page 169)

Torso Twist I and II (pages 153–155)

- Stand in Five-Pointed Star (page 182). Look down to make sure your right foot points forward and your left foot is turned out about 45 degrees.

- Both arms are out to the sides, parallel to floor. Your torso forms a T. Buckle your seat belt. Exhale . . . and reach your right hand out to the right, as though sliding your arm across the kitchen counter.

- Then drop your right hand to your right shin, just below your knee, or place it on a block that's resting on the outside of your right foot. If your right leg feels tight and uncomfortable, repeat Hug a Tree.

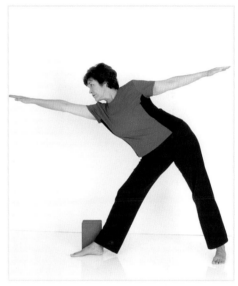

- Lift and reach your left arm. Look up at your left hand. Try pulling both hands away from each other. Extend the sides of your torso parallel to the floor. Keep breathing. Smile . . . this is meant to be fun!

YIN TIP: *Bend your right knee slightly if your leg still feels tight. Look down to the floor if your neck hurts.*

- Come up slowly and repeat two times on each side, then hold the final step for six to eight breaths. Repeat the sequence on the left side.

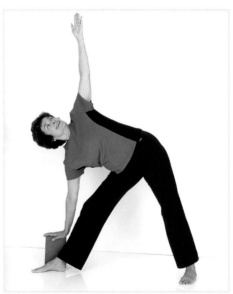

WARRIOR I POSE (*VIRABHADRASANA*)

The reference to "warrior" in this pose does not suggest aggression as a solution to our problems. Here, "warrior" refers to both men and women. It is taken from the Tibetan Pawo, which means "one who is brave." The key to being this warrior is not being afraid of who you are. Ultimately, this is the definition of bravery, of being fearless at knowing yourself—and understanding that it is possible to be heroic and kindly at the same time. This is ahimsa (nonviolence) in action.

USE THE FOLLOWING WARMUPS:

Salutation to the Hips, part or all (page 216)

Victory Goddess (page 77)

Frog Pose (page 115)

Triangle Pose (page 181)

Fan Pose (page 176)

BENEFITS: *Strengthens legs and pelvic muscles; improves balance and posture; brings mobility to shoulders and opens the chest.*

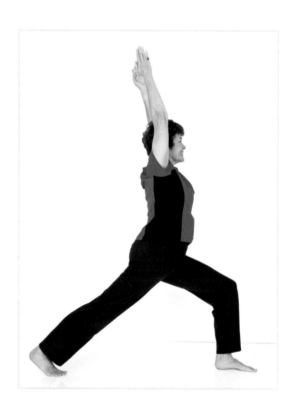

- Stand in Five-Pointed Star. Rotate your left foot out 90 degrees, and turn your right foot in 45 degrees. Turn your pelvis so it faces squarely over your left leg. Raise your right heel slightly off the floor. Inhaling, raise your arms overhead, palms facing each other. Relax your shoulders. Draw your seat-belt muscles inward. Lift your chest away from the waist. Exhaling, bend your left knee so it's over your toes. Look down. Is your knee aligned over your foot? Try not to lean forward.

- Hold the pose for three to six breaths. Sense the soaring upward energy of the arms and the downward grounding energy of the earth. Don't overdo it. Gaze forward, or look upward between your hands into infinity.

- Come out of the pose. Inhaling, straighten your left leg. Return your feet to center in Five-Pointed Star. Repeat the Warrior steps on the opposite side. Then rest in Fan Pose (page 176).

WARRIOR II POSE

Yin Tip: Rolling your inner thighs outward is an important subtlety to this pose. It releases your pelvis and gives freedom to your pose.

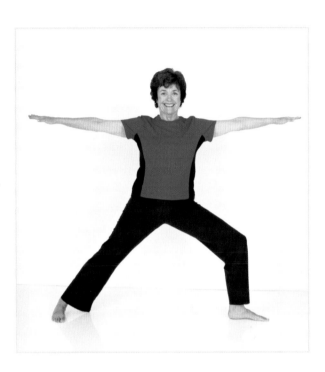

- Stand in Five-Pointed Star. Look down at your feet . . . left foot out at a 90-degree angle, right foot in at 45 degrees. Bend your left knee, keeping it over the ankle. Right leg is straight, its little toe pressed to the floor. Inhaling, raise both arms into a T. Open the eyes of your heart and buckle seat belt. Your spine is long and centered over your hips. Roll your thighs outward. Exhaling, imagine energy extending through your arms and beyond your fingertips.

- Turning your head and holding for two or three breaths can relax neck tension. Hold the posture for five or six breaths. Repeat on the opposite side. Then rest in Fan Pose (page 176).

- You can also practice this pose with your right foot pressing against a wall. This helps your thigh to roll outward. If you keep your right hand on the wall, it will help your torso to be centered over your hips.

EXTENDED SIDE ANGLE POSE (*UTTHITA PARSAVAKONASANA*)

BENEFITS: *Increases strength and flexibility of thighs, legs, hips, and back. Very energizing, it opens the chest! Lateral stretch for rib cage.*

- Stand in Mountain Sacred Pose (page 174). Center yourself. Exhaling, bring palms together in Namaste. Step your feet apart. Go into Five-Pointed Star, with arms in a T.

- Look at your feet. Turn your left foot inward (at about a 45-degree angle), right foot outward (90-degree angle). Inhaling, let your breath fill your body to the tips of your fingers and toes.

- Exhaling, bend your right knee to form a right angle. Rest your right forearm on that knee. Look down to see that your right knee is over your right ankle. Try not to sag into your right shoulder. Instead, press downward into your right forearm, lifting out of your shoulder. Bring your left arm up and close to your left ear, palm down.

- Buckle seat belt. Inhale; lift your rib cage away from your waist. Peek under your left armpit as you reach with enthusiasm outward with your left hand. Hold for at least 30 seconds, three to six breaths.

- Come out of the posture. Return to Five-Pointed Star and repeat these steps on the opposite side.

- Variation: Place the block along the inside of your right foot. Instead of leaning on your thigh, reach down and place your right hand on the block. As you progress, remove the block and place your hand to the floor.

YIN TIP: *Resting in Fan Pose, elbows crossed, feels wonderful after Extended Side Angle Pose!*

USE THE FOLLOWING WARMUPS:

Rolling Pin Series (pages 74–75)

Torso Twist I and II (pages 153–155)

Hug a Tree (page 68)

Triangle Pose (page 181)

Downward-Facing Dog with Chair (page 69)

Fan Pose (page 176)

Chest Expander (page 52)

Half Moon Balance (page 188)

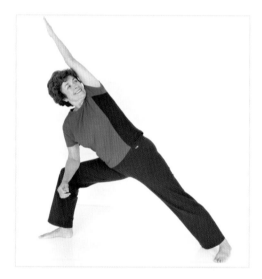

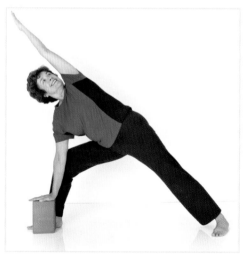

Balancing Poses

Balancing poses are invigorating and refreshing for all ages and levels of ability. They safely challenge your "wobble" muscles—those little muscles you used while learning to ride a bike. Today, they can help you improve your golf swing, stand on a ladder, or even get in and out of a bathtub. It's good to "wobble" in balance poses. Those little muscles will get stronger and stronger with regular practice. Balancing poses help remove the aches and pains of aging, improve mobility and circulation, and strengthen your confidence.

TREE SERIES (*VRKSASANA*)

BENEFITS: *Improves balance and coordination. My students report that practicing balancing poses like Tree awakens awareness of keeping balance in their daily lives.*

USE THE FOLLOWING WARMUPS:

Dancing the Star (page 113)

Stargazing Situp (page 48)

Downward-Facing Dog with Chair (page 69)

STAGE ONE: LOW TREE POSE

- Begin by standing near a wall or a sturdy chair in case you need extra support. Remind yourself to maintain good posture while in Tree Pose. Stand tall in Sacred Mountain Pose (page 174), feet rooted to the earth.

- Shift your weight onto your left foot, and place your right heel on top of the arch of your left foot, laying the right foot softly over the left. This is the low foot position.

- Place your hands together in Namaste. Buckle your seat belt to stabilize the posture. Stand tall . . . breathe . . . gaze at the floor in front of you, finding your balance. Hold for three to six breaths. Repeat on the opposite foot.

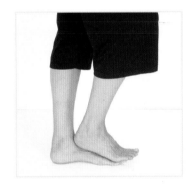

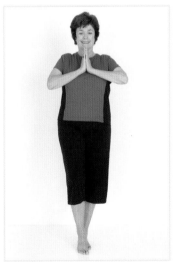

continued on page 186

STAGE TWO: HIGH TREE

● Stand tall in Sacred Mountain Pose, feet rooted to the earth.

● Shift your weight to your left foot. Bend your right knee and place
the foot at the top of your left inner thigh, or as high as you can
comfortably reach. (You can use your hands on your right ankle
to help you place your foot properly.) Press your right knee back;
otherwise, it will naturally want to creep forward. Buckle up that
seat belt! Your gaze is softly focused in front of you.

● Place your palms together in Namaste. Hold pose. Are you having
fun yet? Repeat on the opposite leg.

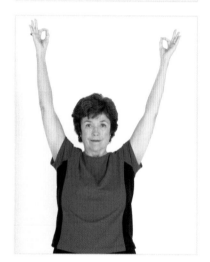

STAGE THREE: CHANGING TREE

*Practice Tree (both high and low poses) with awareness of your mind-
body-spirit connection. In a moment, you are going to experience the
four seasons as they are happening within you, so much so that you will
feel their coming and passing within your tree-body. Each season will
carry a personal message.*

YIN TIP: *Read the directions over completely, pausing at the ellipses.
You could also speak the directions into a tape recorder and play them
back.*

● What sort of tree would you like to be? Choose the leaves, the size
and shape . . . now, stand as that tree . . . either low- or high-foot
position. Feel the clarion call of the coming of spring . . . extend
your arms, your leafy branches, straight up, palms facing inward
but relaxed. Join your thumb and index finger . . . new life
growing . . . budding . . . greening . . . coming to be . . .

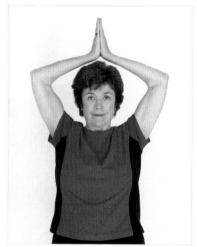

● Now feel the rolling in of summer . . . place your palms together
like a hot flame over your head . . . the heat . . . and ripening . . . the sultry sensuousness of summer.

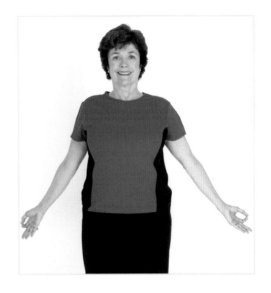

- And now . . . the arrival of autumn . . . let your arms fall out from your body, thumb and index finger together . . . there is lightness after the heavy heat of summer . . . the air surrounds you with crispness . . . vitality . . .

- And after that . . . feel the coming on of winter . . . place your palms together in front of your chest in Namaste . . . the symbol of quiet closure . . . endings . . . maturity . . . cold and dying . . . knowing your own dying . . .

- And then . . . finally . . . once again . . . it is spring . . . raise both arms joyfully above your head again . . . with the spring comes . . . rebirth . . . hope in the sense that all of life renews itself . . . feelings of surging youth . . . the certainty that life continues . . . feel it now . . . keenly in your body . . . mind . . . spirit . . . . Now, return both feet to the floor . . . lower your arms. Take a moment to absorb the four seasons, then repeat on the opposite leg. With practice, you will know all of this and much more . . . and you will know it fully.

HALF MOON BALANCE (*ARDHA CHANDRASANA II*)

BENEFITS: *Develops balance and concentration; improves coordination; strengthens legs and seat muscles; frees and opens rib cage and shoulders and, thus, improves breathing.*

YIN TIP: *Have your blocks ready. Practice Half Moon at the wall at first, then graduate to the center of the room. Triangle Pose (page 181) is a good preparation for Half Moon Balance. Be comfortable with Triangle before trying this one.*

USE THE FOLLOWING WARMUPS:

Salutation to the Hips, all or part (page 216)

Frog Pose (page 115)

Downward-Facing Dog with Chair (page 69)

Tree Series (pages 185–187)

Victory Goddess (page 77)

- Stand in Sacred Mountain Pose. Center yourself . . . eyes soft, gaze inward, watch the breath flowing effortlessly in and out. Palms together in Namaste.

- Go into Five-Pointed Star. Raise your arms out to the sides to form a T, and take a big step left (about one leg's length apart).

- Turn both feet to the right, left foot in 45 degrees and right foot out at about a 90-degree angle. Inhale.

- Exhale and stretch into Triangle Pose. Place your block slightly in front of your right big toe.

- Now move into Half Moon. Look down to the floor. Bend your right knee . . . lean forward and place your right hand on the floor (or a block) about a foot away from your right foot. Lean into your right hand. Place your left hand on your lower back. Your left foot will leave the floor slightly. You are now balanced on your right foot and hand.

- Keep the right knee slightly bent. Inhaling, raise your left leg up in line with your torso, so your body is now parallel to the floor. Exhaling, keep your right knee soft as you slowly press

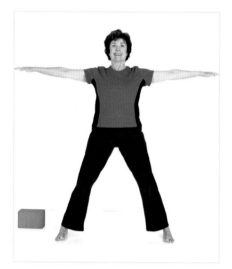

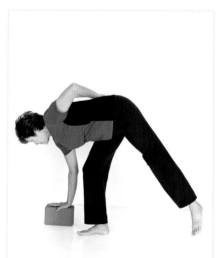

your right leg straight. Root your right foot and toes into the earth. Lengthen your right arm with your inhalation . . . rotate your chest upward as you exhale. Gaze is downward.

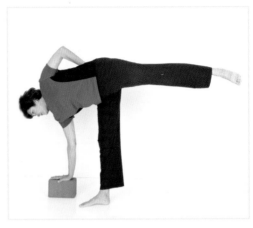

- Take a moment to feel your body in this pose. Feel its shape. Steady the balance. Keep breathing. With practice you'll feel more and more comfortable. As you lengthen your right arm, lift your torso upward. The higher the lift, the easier it is to rotate your chest.

- Finally, lift your left arm slowly up to the sky. Pull your hands away from each other. Move your gaze from the floor to the side. Go slowly. It's tricky.

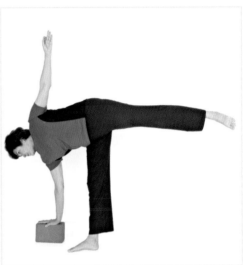

- Come out of the pose as beautifully as you went into it. Bend your right knee. Place your left foot to the floor. Bring your right hand to the ankle. Inhale, straighten your right leg, and slowly stand back up into the Five-Pointed Star.

- Lower your arms. Turn your feet straight. Pause a moment to enjoy. Savor how the posture feels in your body. Then repeat all these steps on your opposite side.

LUNGE POSE (*ASHWA SANCHALASANA*)

Another personal favorite. Everyone can do this pose in one form or another. Have your blocks handy. In Lunge, you will gain insight into your areas of hip and leg tightness. I teach this lunge in levels. It will lead you into many interesting variations and creative posture flows.

LEVEL ONE

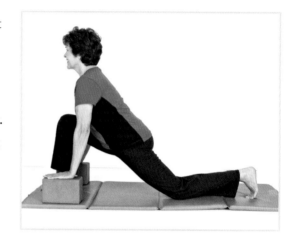

- Begin on your knees. Lean forward and place your left hand to the mat for balance. Then, reach back with your right hand, lift and guide your right leg out . . . around . . . and now in front of you. Place both hands on blocks on either side of your right foot. Look down. Be sure your right knee is over your right ankle. Secure in this position . . . turn your back toes under and inch-slide your back knee further behind you. Knees stay on the mat. Pause here . . . take a breather . . . turning the back toes under will take weight off the knee.

- Exhaling, try to slowly straighten your back leg without letting your hips rise. At first, this will be challenging, but after doing the three Rs, everything will feel easier. Hold for two to four breaths. Return both knees to the floor and repeat all the steps of level one, using the opposite leg. Use the three Rs to release tight muscles in the front and back of your leg.

LEVEL TWO

- Repeat the steps of level one. Now, with your hands on the blocks or on the floor, Resist . . . push your right foot firmly into the mat, and press your hands into the surface with a steady, gentle pressure. Observe the muscles in your front leg contracting. Hips stay down . . . hold resistance steady and even for three breaths . . . Relax . . . breathe in . . . exhaling, Re-stretch. Straighten the back leg . . . your hips and thigh muscles release . . . notice you are able to lower your hips with ease. Gradually remove the blocks. Release . . . and repeat levels one and two on the opposite leg.

HEART LUNGE VARIATION

Though this pose is an important part of connecting with the bliss body (see chapter 16), it's also important to do the Heart Lunge Variation as part of your routine.

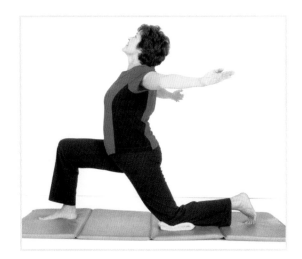

- Come into Lunge position, but this time modify it by aligning your back (left) knee with your left hip. The knee stays on the mat or on a folded towel. Be sure your right knee is in line with your ankle and not out past your foot. Lift your chest until your spine is vertical. Extend your arms out to form a T, palms up . . . in the gesture of giving. Arch your spine comfortably, and buckle your seat belt. Pull your arms back, closing the gates of the shoulders. Inhaling, look up, and lift up your heart. Exhaling, give away your love today . . . to your family . . . to those in need . . . to all beings. No matter how much love you give away, there is always plenty for all. Hold the pose for three to six breaths.

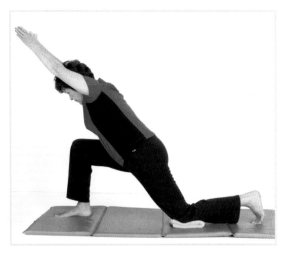

- Receive love today. Keep your modified Lunge stand. Round your back, slowly move your arms out of the T, and bring them forward, up near your ears, rib cage to thigh. Press your palms together, pull fingers away, drop chin to throat . . . head bows in gratefulness. Hold, lengthening the spine, reaching with the fingertips, for 30 seconds. In your mind and heart, receive love today. Repeat the first step. Again, give your love away. Repeat the second step . . . receive love today.

- Repeat Heart Lunge on the opposite leg. Then sit quietly. Close your eyes. Feel the posture and thoughts of giving and receiving love vibrating within your body.

Inversion Postures

Of all the different yoga postures, inverting your body each day is perhaps the most effective in influencing an overall change in your body and mind. Inversion simply means you lift your legs above your heart, using the force of gravity to improve blood flow back to the heart. For thousands of years, yoga masters knew that by tricking gravity with the help of inversions, you can reverse and soften the effects of aging, improve your health, and add years to your life. When you practice yoga, you systematically place various parts of your body both above and below the level of your heart, refreshing the blood supply to each area.

LEGS-UP-ON-THE-WALL POSE (*VIPARITA KARANI*)

BENEFITS: *Calms the nervous system. Improves circulation throughout the body. Restores and rebuilds energy reserves and helps quiet hot flashes in women and prostatitis in men.*

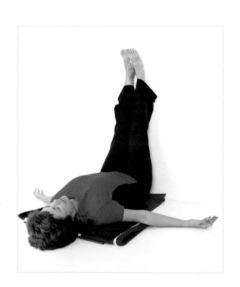

- Sit sideways, with your right hip a few inches away from the wall, legs extended forward.

- Exhaling, swing both legs up the wall and lie down flat on your back, shoulders on the floor. If it's more comfortable, place folded blankets beneath your hips.

- Extend your legs up the wall as far as comfortably possible . . . arms are out to your sides, palms up or down. Place an eye pillow or cloth across your eyes, or simply close them. Relax . . . observe the rise and fall of your breathing. Heart and chest are open, spacious. Hold for 5 minutes. As you stay in the pose, the agitation and fatigue that often accompany stress will fad away.

- Come out slowly. Bring your knees to your chest. Roll over onto your right side. Make a pillow out of your right arm. This is Seed Pose. A transition moment . . . rest for half a minute. Then lean forward, place your left hand on the floor in front of your chest, and slowly come up. Turn and sit with your back against the wall. Close eyes. Dive inward. Enjoy the stillness for a little longer.

HALF SHOULDERSTAND (*SALAMBA SARVANGASANA*)

BENEFITS: *Each of the Shoulderstand variations provides common benefits: improved circulation to the legs, hips, back, neck, heart, and head. I like visualizing the lines of my face softening as old, dead cells wash away in this inverted pose. This posture stimulates endocrine glands and improves lymphatic drainage. It rests in the heart, and calms and rejuvenates the nervous system.*

USE THE FOLLOWING WARMUPS:

Chest Expander (page 52)

Spider on the Wall (pages 204–205)

Stargazing Situp (page 48)

Bridge Pose (page 156)

Cobra Pose (pages 162–163)

Salutation to the Moon (page 218)

YIN TIP: *Use the wall at first. It can really help you gain control and awareness. And remember that even legs up a chair or a wall contain many of the same benefits.*

CAUTION: *The upper neck is vulnerable and needs to be prepared with dynamic (moving) postures, like Bridge and Cobra poses. Do not attempt these inverted poses if you have unmedicated high blood pressure or a hiatal hernia, are moderately overweight, or have glaucoma or neck problems. Come down out of the pose if you need to sneeze, cough, or yawn.*

- Neatly fold two firm blankets and place them on the floor, next to a sturdy (non-mirrored!) wall. Prepare them in a way so that when you swing your feet to the wall in the next step, you'll lie back with the two folded blankets supporting you from your shoulders all the way down to your hips. Your head will rest on the floor. Sit sideways to the wall with your knees bent.

- Now lie on your back, feet flat to floor, heels at your seat, toes touching the base of the wall.

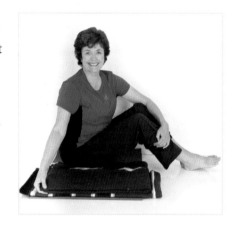

- Place your soles on the wall until your knees form a right angle—thighs parallel, and shins perpendicular, to the wall. Your arms remain at your sides, on the blankets. At this point, you and your blanket might want to scoot closer or farther away to get the angle just right. The blanket acts like a platform to lift and support your vertebrae.

continued on page 194

- Inhaling, press down into the blankets with your hands, push your feet into the wall, and lift your hips comfortably high. Your neck remains soft. At this point lift your hips and roll your spine slowly up and down off the mat, bringing some dynamic warmup movement to this pose.

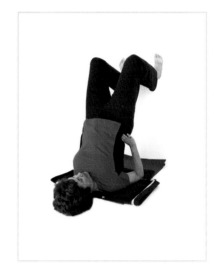

- Bend your elbows, lift your hips higher, and slide your hands up to support your lower back. Press your elbows and backs of arms into the floor to create lift, space, and support. Be sure your shoulders remain on the blanket and the back of your head stays on the floor. Relax your neck—no pain or pressure. Stay here for half a minute and breathe.

- Exhaling, take one foot off wall and extend the leg until you are looking straight up to see the tip of your big toe.

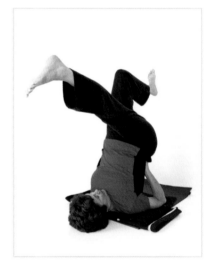

- Try one leg at a time, or raise both legs. Alternate legs, dividing time evenly between each leg. Stay in this step for as long as you are comfortable. Work up to holding the pose for 1 minute or longer. Do your yoga breathing.

- To come down, slowly place one foot, then the other, back on the wall, finally lowering your hips to the floor. Rest in Legs-Up-the-Wall for a minute longer. Then, to come out of this pose, turn on to your right side, in Seed Pose, knees to chest. Right arm makes a pillow. Rest.

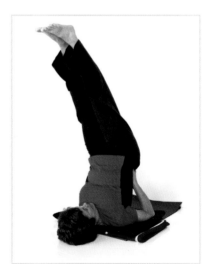

YIN TIP: *In the beginning, it is normal to feel a little tightness in your back when you come out of Half Shoulderstand. Rest in Knees to Chest (page 62), and it should be gone in minutes.*

RELAXATION: SPONGE POSE (SAVASANA)

This pose is also called Long Relaxation (see chapter 7) or Corpse Pose.

BENEFITS: *With regular practice, 5 minutes of relaxation will help you heal the effects of chronic stress. The nervous system sends and receives fewer messages and becomes quieter. Layers of tension, known and unknown, melt away. You learn to stay present and focused on what's going on in your body and mind, from moment to moment.*

- Lie on your back, covered with a blanket so that you are comfortably warm. You may place small pillows or rolled towels beneath your head and knees to relieve tension. If you like, cover your eyes with a cloth or eye pillow.
- Close your eyes, because when the outer eyes are closed, the inner eyes begin to open. Now feel where your upper lid touches your lower lid. When you focus on your eyes, your brain waves quiet down.

- Still with eyes closed, watch your breath as it flows through your nose . . . quiet . . . shallow . . . easy breathing. Notice your breath is cool as it flows in and warm as you breathe out.
- Now focus your attention down to your chest, and watch your breath rise and fall in your chest. Natural breathing, no technique. Nowhere to go, nothing to do, your breath flows comfortably in, and effortlessly out.
- Now bring your awareness down to your feet (focus), and feel where your heels connect to the surface. Silently *suggest* to yourself, "my heels touch," then *pause*. Now *feel* where your heels touch.
- Now slowly bring your awareness to your calves . . . thighs . . . seat muscle. Pause. Feel where your seat muscle touches the surface.
- Continue moving your awareness up to the arch of your low back, into your shoulders, then elbows. Now *focus* your attention like a narrow beam of light into your hands and suggest silently, "My fingers are long." *Pause.* Now

continued on page 196

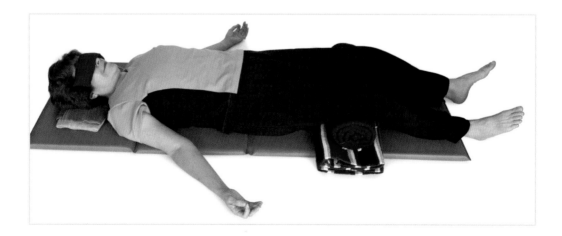

feel the length of your fingers, the space between them, feel sensation, pulsation, warmth in the palms of your hands. Now silently *suggest*, "My hands are empty." *Pause*. Then *feel* the sensation of empty, hollow hands. If you feel nothing, that's fine; just repeat. Feel your hands as empty gloves, lying on your kitchen table. Empty hands.

- Now bring that empty, hollow feeling up through your wrists, elbows, arms, shoulders, up through the busy thoroughfare of your neck. Focus on your eyes. Feel where your eyelids touch. With your eyes closed, look up gently into the lines of your forehead. Feel the little lines between your eyes and your brow that hold small cares and worries. Suggest, "The little lines on my forehead are smooth." Pause. Feel your forehead. Feel the little lines smoothing out, the cares and worries dissolving.

- Now focus on your mouth. Feel where the lips touch. Feel the length of your lips. Now go inside the dark cave of your mouth. Shine the light of your internal focus on your tongue. Feel its length, and the little lake of feeling in the center of your tongue. Now focus your attention on the muscle that hinges the upper jaw to the lower jaw. Silently suggest, "My jaw muscle is slack." Pause. Feel this hinge of the jaw slacken. Feel the open space within your mouth. Feel where the two lips touch.

- Take a moment to gaze downward and observe. Watch your breath as it rises and falls in your chest. Pause. On your next exhale, suggest the word "heavy." Pause to feel your chest. Your ribs are heavy. Again, focus on the chest and suggest "heavy." Feel the bones of your ribs, spine, and shoulders, heavy as steel. Wait to

feel the heaviness. Take your time.

- Now focus your awareness on your breathing as it flows into both nostrils; cool as you breathe in, warm as you breathe out. It's normal if your mind wanders.

- Relax all efforts and dive into the stillness.

- Coming out of relaxation consciously is important. Before you move, scan your body: feel both legs, sense both arms, torso, neck, and head. Feel the whole body. Take an enjoyable yawn.

- Slowly raise arms over your head, stretch one side, stretch another, stretch your whole body.

- Ask yourself, "What can I take with me that is positive into my day? What feelings, what qualities that strengthen, nurture, improve my waking hours or ease me into sleep?"

- Now, slowly rise, feeling rested and refreshed, clear in mind and spacious in body.

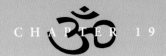

CHAPTER 19

PARTNER WORK

There are many advantages in using a partner (your yoga-slave) for asana practice. The "receiver" (partner 1) can concentrate on sensation and awareness as well as on the details of alignment, observing the posture, and breathing. The "helper" (partner 2) is there to support, check the partner's form, and provide friendly feedback.

It is important to honor your partner's space. Come into it slowly and with respect. You are there to assist, not change, your partner. Injuries can occur when one partner thinks he can change the other or tries to "force" a position. I encourage partners to talk quietly to each other. The "receiver" *must* be in control of the final position, and not the other way around. Listening to your body and being responsible is part of your journey. Self-awareness and respect for your partner cannot be achieved without embracing responsibility.

It simply feels good in our emotional body, our mano-maya-kosha, to be supported by another human being. Working with a partner allows you to experience the subtleties of the asana that can be recaptured when practicing on your own. Go to a hatha class that from time to time does partner work. Find someone close to your size and weight to partner with. Although the opposite can be fun, too!

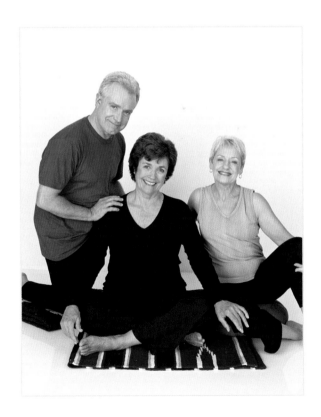

PARTNER HAMSTRING STRETCH (*SUPTA PADANGUSTHASANA*)

STEP ONE

USE THE FOLLOWING WARMUPS:

Rolling Pin Series (pages 74–75)

Seaweed Legs (page 63)

Wall Calf Stretch (page 65)

- Kevin, partner 1 (the receiver), lies on his back, left leg bent so the left foot is on the floor. He extends his right leg up toward the ceiling as straight as possible, with his foot flexed.

- Nancy, partner 2 (the helper), kneels or stands behind Kevin's right leg. She tests the flexibility of his hamstring by holding on to his right heel and gently pressing it away from her (toward Kevin) until they both feel the first point of resistance.

- As the receiver of this exercise, you are relaxed. Do not force anything. Listen to your body, and tell your partner when you are close to the edge of sweet discomfort (not pain).

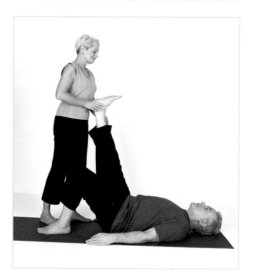

STEP TWO

- Now the three Rs. Nancy takes a wider stance, bending her knees for support. She guides Kevin's right leg back to the starting point, then begins the Resistance. She places one hand on top of his foot, and gently pushes her other hand into his right heel. She holds for three to five breaths (10 seconds).

- Kevin begins the Resistance. He pushes his heel gently and steadily back into Nancy's hand, ignoring the urge to bounce. (This Resistance will not work if you bounce.) He holds for three to five breaths (10 seconds).

- After holding for 10 seconds, Kevin Relaxes his whole body, breathes in, and on the exhale, Nancy Restretches his leg.

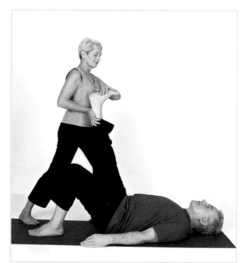

STEP THREE

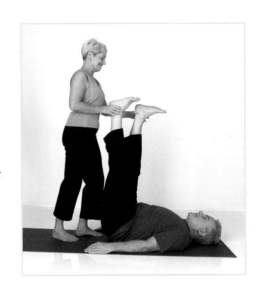

- For this part, Nancy goes very, very slowly. She lets Kevin feel the fibers lengthen and encourages him to breathe, relax, feel, and enjoy this painless and wonderful way to stretch the hams. This can be held for 1 minute.

YIN TIP: *At this point, it's very interesting to see how far you've come. Nancy holds the right leg at its comfortable maximum stretch position. Kevin raises his left leg up to the ceiling to its natural stopping point. Look at the difference in legs! I hope you'll feel encouraged that you can improve your flexibility today (not in 3 months' time), and it will last with practice.*

- Repeat steps one through three on the opposite leg. Then Nancy and Kevin will switch roles. Knowing how the stretch feels will help Kevin give back to Nancy.

PARTNER TORSO TWIST (*SUPTA MATSYENDRASANA*)

CAUTION: *You should have full knowledge of the Torso Twist poses before attempting Partner Torso Twist.*

- Partner 1, Nancy, lies down and goes through the beginning steps of Torso Twist II. Once she's in the final position, she asks her partner, Kevin, to kneel beside her, as in the photo.

- Kevin kneels beside Nancy with his down knee close to her hips, near her sacrum (tailbone area). He places his near hand on her hip, and the other hand on her extended arm, just above her elbow (not her shoulder—that's too uncomfortable). Kevin lean his weight evenly into Nancy's extended arm and hip. Once in position, they begin the three Rs.

- Nancy pushes her top hip back into Kevin's hand for a few breaths. This begins the Resistance. She need not push hard—if Kevin cannot hold her in position, she's pushing too hard. After pushing back gently, she Relaxes . . . breathes in . . . exhales . . . then slowly guides her own knee closer to the floor with her nonextended hand.

- Ask your partner to hold you in this new position for about 5 to 10 breaths. Close your eyes, and enjoy this amazing stretch. Release slowly . . . return to the center of your mat, and repeat all the steps on the opposite side.

USE THE FOLLOWING WARMUPS:

Standing, Ring the Gong (page 55)

Standing, Fill the Cup (page 76)

Standing Forward Bend with BLock,
   Alternating Legs (page 61)

If front of arms and chest are tight:

Spidey on the Mat (page 71)

Partner Spider on the Wall (pages 204–205)

Torso Twist I and II (pages 153–155)

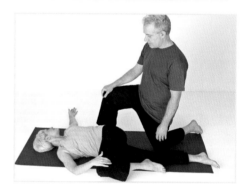

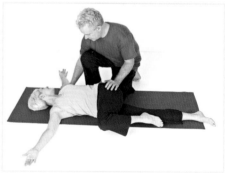

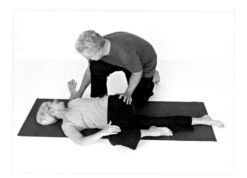

PARTNER SUSPENSION BRIDGE (UTKATASANA)

- Stand face-to-face, clasping your partner's wrists. Step back, arm's-length away, engaging all the arm muscles. With your feet hip-width apart, fold forward from your hips. Now pull back from the hips. Talk to your partner: do you need more pull or less? Hold for three or four breaths.

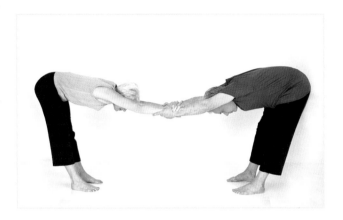

- Walk your feet forward, and bend at the knees as though sitting in a chair. Bring your ribs to your thighs, and pull back from the hips. Hold for three or four breaths.

- To come out of Suspension Bridge, keep tension on the arms, bend your elbows, and then straighten up.

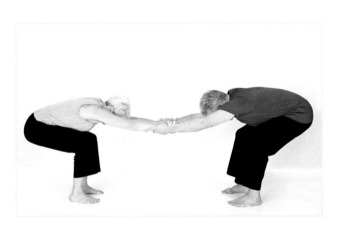

PARTNER-ASSISTED CHEST EXPANDER (*YOGA MUDRA*)

BENEFITS: *This posture rewards you with most of the same benefits as the solo Chest Expander, described on page 52. However, this posture can be deepened when you work with a partner. The three Rs work beautifully with Chest Expander. It is the perfect warmup for Cobra Pose (pages 162–163), Camel Pose (pages 150–151), and Half Shoulderstand (pages 193–194).*

REMINDER: *When working in pairs, one of you is there to support the other. Go slowly; do not push your partner into overextending. Speak gently and quietly to each other.*

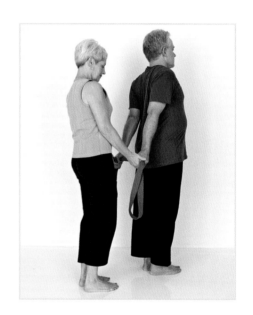

- Kevin, partner 1 (the receiver), begins by warming up his shoulders with shoulder rolls forward and backward, and spider hands on the wall or floor.

- Kevin stands and clasps a belt behind him. His palms face his seat muscle, and his arms are straight. He rolls his shoulders back and down before continuing. This is essential! Nancy, partner 2 (the helper), comes behind and places her hands on Kevin's wrists or under his knuckles to hold his arm positions steady.

- Now Kevin does the three Rs by pressing his hands down toward floor, deepening the back and down position of his shoulders. His arms do not move, however. Nancy helps him hold the steady Resistance.

  Talk to your partner if you are not getting enough support (or too much), causing you to push too hard. Hold the contraction for eight to ten breaths—then *stop* . . . Relax . . . breathe in . . . out . . . then Restretch.

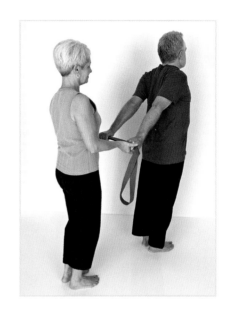

- Nancy slowly . . . very, very slowly . . . lifts and guides Kevin's arms up. Talking to each other, they come to the edge of what feels comfortable and strong. No pain! Kevin breathes in fully, lifts his chest . . . buckle his seat belt. On the next exhale . . . maybe lift a bit higher . . . release.

- Now Nancy helps guide Kevin's arms down slowly. Then he lets go of the belt and closes his eyes, observing the lightness in his arms and shoulders.

YIN TIP: *The closer your hands are together, the more intense the arm and shoulder stretch. Open the eyes of your heart.*

CAUTION: *Don't sacrifice movement in the shoulder joint for the sake of more arm height. The most common error in this pose is to bend forward so you can raise your arms higher.*

Partner Spider on the Wall

Benefits: *Very effective stretch for the biceps, the muscle between the crook of your elbow and your shoulder. We don't think of this little muscle as being tight. However, a tight biceps affects many postures (Downward-Facing Dog especially) and can cause soreness and irritation in the elbow and shoulder. Spider will help your golf swing!*

Yin Tip: *We'll do Spider on the Wall in stages. Go slowly and cautiously, especially if you have had shoulder injuries.*

STAGE ONE

- Kevin, partner 1 (the receiver), faces a wall and places his left arm, extended, against it. His hand is above his shoulder level, and his thumb is turned up. He places his right hand on the wall for support. Nancy, partner 2 (the helper), guides Kevin's arm into position by placing her right hand on the upper part of his left arm and her left hand on the lower part of his arm.

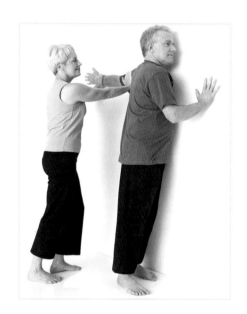

STAGE TWO

- Now Nancy lightly cups her left hand on Kevin's left shoulder, and her right hand on his right shoulder, to help hold it in position. Kevin, keeping his left shoulder to the wall, *slowly* rotates his whole body, using his feet so that his right shoulder comes away from the wall. His right hand helps him to hold the position.

- He should feel the comfortable stretch across the front of his chest, left shoulder, and biceps. Nancy should remind Kevin to move in tiny increments and not lean forward, which would impede the stretch.

- The three Rs can make Spider on the Wall very effective. While Nancy holds Kevin in position, he creates soft Resistance by pressing his palm and wrist (or his extended arm) gently into the wall. He holds for two or three breaths . . . using a slow, long, pushing action . . . he pauses . . . Relaxes . . . breathes in and out . . . Restretches. Very slowly, he rotates his chest away from the wall . . . The receiver must be in control of this final stretch. The helper follows the receiver's move away from the wall and holds the receiver in the new position.

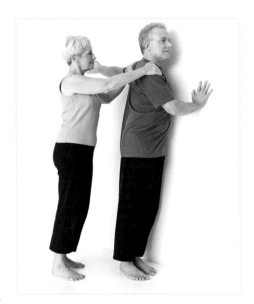

- It's very important that Nancy is guiding this move and not pushing Kevin. Her holding Kevin in the final position truly helps him to concentrate on the sensation in his arm, extend his breathing, and consciously let the fibers of the muscles soften and relax.

- As the receiver, or partner 1, when you come to the comfortable edge of the stretch, deliberately breathe in. Exhaling, relax once more. Observe that you can take yourself a tiny bit further into the stretch.

- To come out of Spider, Nancy guides Kevin's left arm down . . . with no help from him. He pauses here, noticing any differences between the left and right arms. The stages are repeated with the opposite arm.

PARTNER TREE POSE (*VRKSASANA*)

- Stand tall, side by side, with your hips 1 to 2 inches apart.

- Both partners bend their outside leg, placing the soles of their outside feet on the inside of their own thighs, just above their knees. If it's more comfortable, place your foot below your knee. Buckle up your seat belt.

- Intertwine the inside arms, like branches of a tree, and raise them up over your heads.

- Reach with your outside arms across your chests, bringing palms together in Namaste.

- Now let your inside hips touch. Spread the roots of your toes deeply into the earth, standing straight and tall. If you fall out of your tree, try again. Repeat on the opposite sides.

USE THE FOLLOWING WARMUPS:

Low Tree (solo) (page 185)

High Tree (solo) (page 186)

Salutation to the Hips, all or part (page 216)

Frog Pose (page 115)

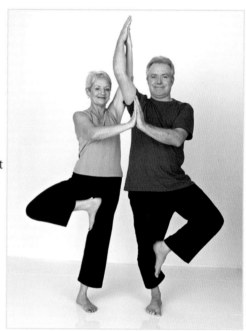

PARTNER SEATED SIDE BEND (*PARIGHASANA*)

BENEFITS: *Excellent stretch for all muscles of the side trunk. Adds ease and grace to Triangle Pose (page 181) and all standing or seated side poses.*

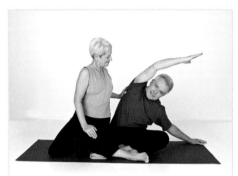

- Kevin, partner 1 (the receiver), sits with his legs folded, his right ankle in front of the left. He has placed a roll beneath his right thigh because it did not meet the floor. While sitting, Nancy, partner 2 (the helper), slides her hip gracefully up, and rests her thigh across Kevin's to hold his hip to the floor. (This move usually evokes a giggle!)

- Nancy places a hand under Kevin's shoulder, assisting him to hold this position steady. The three Rs can improve the final position dramatically. Kevin leans left, with his left hand on the floor. He pushes gently back into Nancy's hand, using his waist and back muscles to press into the Resistance. He holds for a few breaths. Relaxes . . . breathes in . . . exhales . . . Kevin must move into the Restretch himself by extending his top arm out, leaning forward slightly, and letting himself go further to the side. Nancy uses her hand to guide (not push) Kevin as he goes deeper into the pose. She reminds him to relax his shoulders. He holds for three to six breaths, then comes up slowly. Repeat on opposite side.

PARTNER SINGLE LEG FORWARD BEND (*PASCHIMOTTANASANA*)

A partner can really help you deepen and feel this posture.

- Nancy, partner 1 (the receiver), begins by warming up with Seated Forward Bend (page 172).

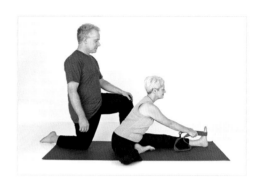

- She now extends her left leg out and places her right foot high on the inside of her left thigh. Leaning forward, she loops her belt around her left foot, which is flexed. She sits up slowly until her back is straight, letting the belt slide through her fingers, while keeping tension on it. Her arms and shoulders are relaxed.

- She's now ready to begin folding forward. Sitting tall, arching her back slightly, her sit bones go back as she slowly folds forward, trying to keep her back straight. There will come a natural stopping place where the spine begins to round. She holds for three to six breaths.

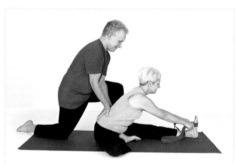

- While Nancy is stretching, Kevin, partner 2 (the helper), kneels behind her. Looking at Nancy's back, he places his hands on the roundest part, which is probably just above her waist. Nancy should be focusing her attention on where Kevin's hands touch her back. This is exactly where a stronger straightening effort is exerted, using the three Rs.

- The three Rs work very effectively in this partner work (though they can also be done in the solo version). Kevin kneels behind Nancy with his hands just above her lower back, right in the curve, just above her waist. Nancy, feeling the support of Kevin's hands and hearing his encouragement to lengthen her back, slowly lifts up her chest and presses back into his hands. Her sit bones slide back, helping her to arch her spine a tiny bit. This effort will help lengthen the mid and upper back painlessly. Hold this Resistance for 1 minute, gentle and steady. Observe the muscles in use during this hold.

- Now, Nancy creates a little more resistance. Holding on to the belt (or even the outer edge of the foot), she Resists by gently pulling her hands away from her foot, which is flexed. Now two actions are going on—she's pulling away from her feet, and she's pressing back into Kevin's hands. Her body stays very still. She holds for 10 breaths, as large muscles benefit from longer contractions.

- Now, Nancy Relaxes . . . breathes in. Exhaling, she Restretches slowly, pulling her torso forward; her spine and neck are long.

You, the receiver, let go of the belt, and place hands on knees, ankles, or floor. Hold for ten more breaths. Relax and enjoy!

- Very slowly come up to a sitting position. Sit for a moment, eyes closed. Dive inward. For the next few moments, enjoy the inner quietude. Then repeat the above steps with the opposite leg. Thank your partner. Then change positions.

- Variation: For a more intense stretch, you can do the traditional Forward Bend with both legs extended.

PARTNER BIRD OF PARADISE (*PARIVRTTA JAN SIRSASANA*)

BENEFITS: *This fabulous stretch feels wonderful and stretches, like pulled taffy, the layers of fascia in addition to many muscles of the trunk.*

USE THE FOLLOWING WARMUPS:

Partner Torso Twist (page 200)

Partner Seated Side Bend (page 207)

Little Mermaid Series (pages 72–73)

PART ONE

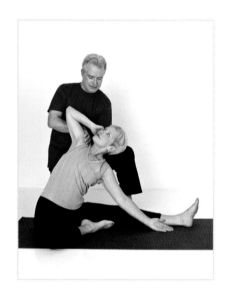

- Nancy, partner 1 (the receiver), sits on the mat, having warmed up well. She extends her left leg toward her left side (not straight out front) and bends her right knee, with her thigh and knee resting on the floor, the sole of her right foot against her left inner thigh. Sitting tall, she turns her torso to the right. Then, leaning to her left, she places her left elbow on the inside of her outstretched leg, resting her hand on the floor, palm up. Her left elbow will press into the side of her leg to help her turn more. Nancy's right hand rests on the back of her head, her elbow pointing toward the ceiling. Kevin, partner 2 (the helper), kneels behind Nancy and places one hand to support her lower shoulder, and uses his other hand to help Nancy roll her top shoulder back, until her shoulders are almost vertical.

- Nancy breathes in. Exhaling, she pulls her held (top) shoulder forward (as Kevin pulls back gently), thus creating a little Resistance, for three breaths. She Relaxes, breathes in, and Restretches, lengthening and revolving on a long exhale. Inhaling, she opens and turns her chest deeper. She is turning her rib cage from her left to her right in this beautiful Bird of Paradise Pose.

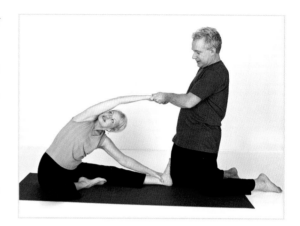

- Now Nancy is in position for part two. She raises her right arm, pulls her right shoulder back, then straightens her arm close to the side of her head. She is now in the full plumage of Bird of Paradise. Kevin helps her deepen the pose. He moves from behind her and kneels at the toes of Nancy's left foot, placing one knee against the bottom of her foot. He reaches and holds on to her outstretched right hand. Her arm is in line with her extended leg.

- For resistance, Nancy tries to slowly pull her right arm back. This little move contracts the side torso muscles. She resists for three to six breaths. Now, she Relaxes . . . breathes in. Kevin helps her, drawing her arm out just a bit further for the Restretch. Nancy, with total focus, revolves and lengthens her torso just a tiny bit more for two or three breaths.

- Come out of this pose slowly. Sit for a moment quietly. Enjoy the finished posture. Repeat on the opposite side.

PARTNER LEAPING FROG POSE (*BHEKASANA*)

BENEFITS: *Frog gives a deep stretch for the inner thighs and hips, making legs more comfortable in meditation and your daily walk.*

CAUTION: *Much of your weight is supported by your arms. If you feel the stretch becoming too strong, use your arms to relieve the stretch immediately. Omit this pose if you have hip or knee challenges. Frog is safe if both partners are sensible and go slowly.*

YIN TIP: *Place a towel beneath each knee so that they will slide easily on the floor. Place a support pillow or folded blanket beneath your chest, if needed.*

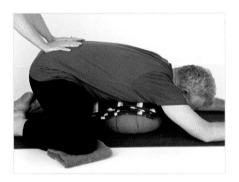

- Kevin, partner 1 (the receiver), lies facedown, well-propped with a blanket and/or pillow under his torso. His legs are pulled up so that his feet are just behind his seat, and his knees are extended outward. Towels are under his knees for comfort. His elbows are comfortably on the mat above his head.

- Nancy, partner 2 (the helper), kneels behind Kevin and places both forearms or hands above his hip joints. No weight is on the curve of his lower back.

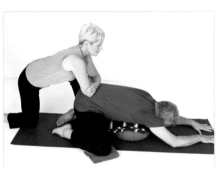

- Now the three Rs. Kevin becomes the Leaping Frog. He tries to squeeze his knees together like a frog trying to leap. Nancy can feel this contraction and holds his hips down with gentle, steady pressure. This creates the Resistance. Hold for six breaths.

- Kevin then Relaxes, breathes in, and exhales. He Restretches. Nancy releases some of her assisted weight, breathes in, then leans a little more weight toward Kevin so he can painlessly and comfortably reach his final Frog stretch. Hold for six to ten breaths.

- After the final Frog stretch, Nancy assists Kevin out of Frog Pose. Kevin does none of this work. Nancy slides his knees slowly straight until he is lying belly-down on the mat. Kevin removes the pillow and relaxes quietly for ten restful breaths.

YIN TIP: *Do not hold Frog longer than 1 minute (even though it's tempting). Too much flexibility in a midlife body can overstretch ligaments that hold the joints in place.*

Partner Happy Baby (*Supta Ekapadasana*)

- Kevin, partner 1 (the receiver), lies flat on the mat. (Place a pillow beneath your head, if needed.) His left leg is straight on the mat. He bends his right knee and places his right hand, or a belt held in his right hand, around his foot. Keeping his knee comfortably bent, he raises his foot toward the ceiling. Nancy, partner 2 (the helper), kneels beside Kevin's outstretched leg. She places her right hand on Kevin's left thigh, above his kneecap. She gently leans into Kevin's left thigh, holding his leg steady. To improve Kevin's position even more, Nancy slides her left hand into the back of Kevin's right leg and gently leans into his leg.

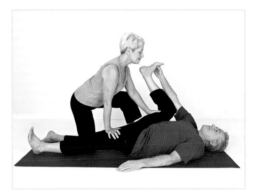

- Now the three Rs. Kevin creates resistance by pushing his right foot into the belt or hand, and at the same time presses his right thigh into Nancy's hand. Yes, this takes concentration. This steady stream of Resistance is held for eight to ten breaths. Nancy talks to Kevin, asking, "Am I pressing too hard or not enough?" She adjusts accordingly, keeping a steady pressure. No bouncing.

- Kevin relaxes . . . breathes in . . . exhales . . . This is the moment when Kevin must Restretch himself in Happy Baby. Note the angle of his right leg in the photo, pressing his right knee toward his armpit. Nancy provides Kevin the helping hands of awareness. Enjoy this moment and hold for 1 minute. Feel the muscles soften and lengthen. No tension anywhere. Release . . . rest a few moments. Repeat on the opposite leg.

- For the more flexible student, open your right knee angle to almost a straight line to increase and deepen hamstring stretch.

Yin Tip: *Some students feel an uncomfortable compression inside the hip. If that happens to you, readjust your clothing, guide your leg, and reposition it further outside the line of your body. Ask your partner to hold you in this new position for ten breaths.*

Partner Moon Breathing and Back-to-Back Twist

Benefits: *Students often observe feelings of anger, nausea, and tears coming up in twists. Please consider this as a positive healing release of negative energy that's buried (sometimes for years) in the muscles and body fascia, as well as in the emotional body,* mano-maya-kosha.

PART ONE

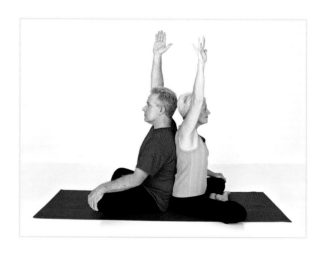

- Partners sit back-to-back, cross-legged, hands on knees, eyes closed. Feel where the two backs touch. Focus on the back of your body. Feel your ribs expanding. Even your tailbone and sacrum move with each breath. Observe for one minute, eyes closed.

- Now explore the mystery of your Moon Breathing. Take your time, eyes still closed. Day-dream of a full moon reflecting its light like a pathway upon the dark ocean. See and feel the waves of breath as they roll in, and slowly out. Observe your breathing in comfortable rhythm with your partner. Continue Moon Breathing for another blissful minute.

PART TWO

- Still sitting back to back, both partners raise the right arm toward the ceiling, fingers up, keeping left hand on your own left knee.

- Now, reach back and place your right hand on your partner's left knee. Inhale, and lengthen your spine. Exhale, twisting your torsos to the right in unison (toward your outstretched arm), and put your left hand on your own right knee. Hold, breathing out for 3 seconds.

- Inhale; return to center. Now, exhaling, wring out your spine in the opposite direction (away from your outstretched arm).

- Now the three Rs. Each partner holds the Resistance for four to six breaths . . . Relax . . . Breathe in . . . Restretch. Spiraling slowly, partners again twist to the right, repeating all the steps. Keep your neck soft, turning your head to the left last. Hold the twist for 30 seconds, breathing comfortably.

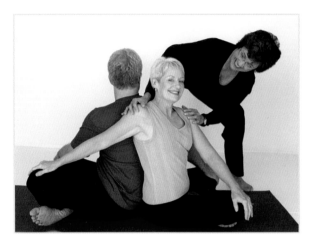

YIN TIP: *Twisting in the opposite direction before the final pose helps release the tight layers of abdominal fascia. Your comfort and ease in the twist will improve with this little move.*

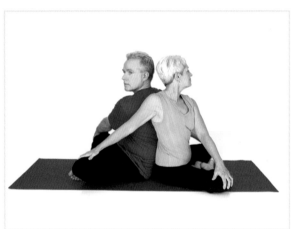

- To finish, come back to center . . . eyes closed . . . enjoy the stillness for 1 minute and repeat part two on the opposite side.

CHAPTER 20

SUGGESTED ROUTINES

The following lists are yoga routines I've put together for you to use when you want to practice yoga for a specific need. For example, you might want a shorter calming practice, an energizing one, or a longer, more intense practice.

While there are countless routines I could compose, these are just a few that flow easily and are not too difficult. The most important requirement: have fun!

SALUTATION TO THE HIPS

- Sit Quietly: Namaste
- Hip Rolls from Rolling Pin Series (pages 74–75)
- Knees to Chest (page 62)
- Dancing the Star (page 113)
- Low Tree Pose (page 185)
- Torso Twist I and II with three Rs (pages 153–155)
- Barn Door: Piriformus Stretch (page 66)
- Happy Baby Pose (page 158)
- Seaweed Legs (page 63)
- Little Mermaid Series (pages 72–73)
- Hamstrings Solo (page 59)

SEATED YOGA VACATION

Do this mini-routine on your next office stretch break. These postures and breathing techniques are perfect for doing at work or at home with a chair.

Time: 5 to 10 minutes

- Yawn with Awareness (page 111)
- Three-Part Breathing (page 87)
- Neck Tilt I and II (page 49)
- Shoulder Preparation for Garuda Arms (page 56)

Now, move your spine in six directions:

- Downward-Facing Dog with a Chair (page 69)
- Arc Back: hold for three to six breaths
- Crescent Moon to the right and to the left: hold each side for three to six breaths (page 179)
- Sage Twist right and left: hold each side for three to six breaths (page 169)

- Caring Breath (page 130)
- Short Let-Go Relaxation (pages 37–38)

SHORT PRACTICE

Keep it simple, but gradually hold each of these poses a little longer, working up to 15 seconds on each side. "Holding" is useful for overcoming agitation of the body and mind, known by yoga masters as Rajasic energy. This practice will take you about 20 to 25 minutes.

- Stargazing Yogoda (page 111)
- Three-Part Breathing, emphasizing long exhales, five to ten breaths (pages 87–88)
- Ring the Gong (page 55)
- Fill the Cup (page 76)
- Standing Forward Bend, three to four times, moving in and out dynamically (page 177)
- Hug a Tree (page 68)
- Triangle Pose (page 181)
- Extended Side Angle Pose (page 184)
- Hero's Twist (page 170)
- Seated Forward Bend (page 172)
- Alternate Nostril Breathing, 2 to 3 minutes (pages 88–89)
- Savasana Relaxation, legs up the wall or on a chair, for 3 minutes (pages 195–196)

WEEKEND WORK-IN (A LONGER PRACTICE)

Please reread the guidelines for the three Rs on page 45, remembering that Resistance is not a red-faced effort. Using the three Rs, repeating postures, and "holding" postures for approximately 30 seconds overcomes heaviness of the body and mind, known by the ancients as Tamasic, or heavy energy. Do all or part of this routine when you have a little more time. You might want to listen to a serenity CD.

- Short Let-Go Relaxation (pages 37–38)
- Upper Neck Curve (ball rolling) (page 46)
- Shoulder Roll (ball rolling) (page 47)
- Salutation to the Hips, all or part (opposite page)
- Knees to Chest (page 62)
- Anchored Boat Pose (page 160)
- Kapalabhati breathing, three or four rounds (pages 89–90)
- Flying Sunbird, hold (page 144)
- Pigeon Pushup (page 145)
- Pigeon II, hold (page 146)
- Chataranga I (page 168)
- Salutation to the Moon, three repetitions (pages 218–219). On the third repetition, hold each pose for three breaths.
- Practice your favorite standing poses (start on page 174).
- Practice your least favorite standing pose.
- Practice one balancing pose (starting on page 185).
- Rest in Child's Pose (page 164)
- Sage Twist (page 169)
- Seated Forward Bend (page 172)
- Kapalabhati breathing (pages 89–90)
- Inner Smile Relaxation (pages 128–129)

SALUTATION TO THE MOON

Having no light of her own, Grandmother Moon reflects the light of the sun. The moon reflects a cool, luminous, energizing quality. Ancients believed gazing at the moon strengthened the blood and the mind. The moon energy alters the water of the earth and within our bodies, allowing our bodies to be in tune with the rhythmic lunar cycles. When we do Salutation to the Moon, we soak up her cool, calming energy. To an extent, we are saluting her positive effect on us.

Salutation to the Moon is a soothing *vinyasa* to do in the evening. (A vinyasa is a series of postures meant to be done in a smooth flow from one to the next.) This 17-posture flow symbolizes the lunar phases of Grandmother Moon. It's nice to do when the moon is visible in the sky. It calms the excess heat of thinking and cools the fire element of the body. I've made up my own names for these postures. Feel free to make up your own variations of Salutation to the Moon. Like the rhythm of the tides created by the moon, this posture-flow builds like a wave and peaks with Cobra Pose, then calms back down as you move through the last pose, repeating some of those you've already done.

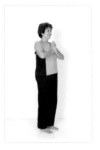

Namaste
to the Moon

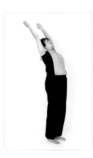

Arc Back

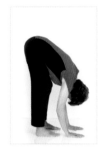

Little Dipper

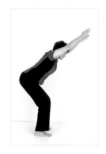

Earth Touch

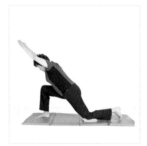

Comet

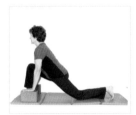

Earth Lunge

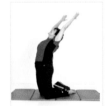

Ascending
Moon

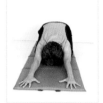

Dark Moon

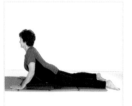

Praying Moon

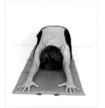

Dark Moon

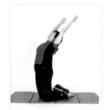

Ascending
Moon

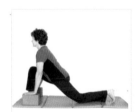

Earth Lunge

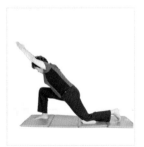

Comet

Earth Touch

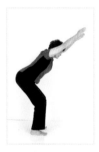

Little Dipper

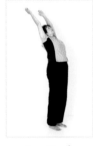

Arc Back

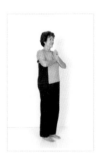

Namaste
to the Moon

CHAPTER 21

SPECIAL CHALLENGES

Illness today is not a simple problem with pat answers. Thousands of studies show that attitude is an important factor in healing. Rather than thinking of illness as an inevitable disaster or unavoidable misfortune, we could think of disease as a useful message to be recognized, acknowledged, and changed.

Doctors throughout the world use relaxation and visualization as ways to revive the nourishing energy that's needed to heal. These techniques produce no side effects and work beautifully and inexpensively with conventional medicine. Holistic physicians and health practitioners worldwide use these tools to help patients recover from surgery or cope with chronic illnesses such as cancer, arthritis, and heart disease. Many of my students have reported that the relaxation techniques they learned in yoga class were tremendously helpful during an MRI or CT scan.

These are some of my thoughts on using yoga as part of your comprehensive plan for healing, regardless of your condition:

▶ No need to expect results quickly; no one is holding a stopwatch.
▶ Let your natural curiosity and interest set your feet upon the path.

▶ You actively participate in your healing journey and become a part of the process.
▶ And when I say "healing," I mean it on many levels: the mind . . . the body . . . the spirit.

A HEALING VISUALIZATION

Visualization-meditation mystics have always valued light as a powerful healing image. To begin, close your eyes and feel a sense of tranquillity in this present moment . . . with your witness at your side . . . daydream . . . remember happy times with candles burning on a dinner table . . . let the image come to you . . . sit in a chair at this table and look at the glowing candle . . . bring the flame closer . . . so that it fills your skull with color and soft warmth . . . Imagine that this light contains the healing powers of the universe . . . wisdom . . . forgiveness . . . love . . . protection . . .

Now radiate this healing light to every cell in your immune system. Radiate this light into a special physical or emotional challenge you have today . . . this light supports and enhances all the medicines you are taking . . . radiate this light out your fingers . . . toes . . . through the top of your head . . . until it surrounds you completely, like a bubble of light . . . now rest in this light for a few more minutes . . . let all the directions and techniques fade away . . . rest . . . giving thanks . . . return to life, refreshed and confident.

"WHEN THE DEEP PURPLE FALLS"—EASE YOURSELF TO SLEEP

There are some people who have difficulty falling asleep because they are still locked into their daytime breathing patterns. If you think this might describe you, try to reestablish your night-time rhythm of breathing. Different practices work for different people. Some folks need to work off restlessness and tense fatigue with some dynamic postures; others sit on the side of their bed and do Caring Breath. Let this relaxation help ease you directly into the sleep state.

Sit at the side of your bed . . . place your right thumb on your forehead, above the eyebrows but below the hairline. This area of your forehead is called the glabella. With your right thumb, lightly stroke from your hairline downward between your eyebrows . . . pause and imagine little cares and worries of the day melting from your glabella. Lie down, knees straight or bent . . . hands on your abdomen . . . continue with slow, easy abdominal breath-ing . . . feel your chest getting heavy on each exhale . . . feel the face muscles relaxing, jaw slack . . . draw your attention deeply inward. Visualize the deep, rich, velvety-purple of nightfall . . . inhaling about 3 seconds . . . exhaling 3 seconds . . . inhaling 3 . . . exhaling 3 . . . body heavy . . . heavy bones . . . feel bones heavy . . . sinking into the mat . . . inhale 3 . . . exhale 3. After a while, turn over on your side . . . pillow between the knees . . . continue inhaling 3 . . . exhaling 3 . . . pull the deep, warm, velvety purple cloak of nightfall over your body as you fall fast asleep.

HINTS FOR SENIORS FOR GETTING UP FROM THE FLOOR

Few experiences are more demoralizing for older adults than falling and not being able to get back up. In my Silver Gentle Moments video series, I specifically spend time showing my older students how to get up from and down on the floor. The time to practice it is *now*, when you don't need it. I assure you it gets easier and easier with practice. Remember the golden rule about most physical activity: Use it or lose it.

1. Stand next to a study chair or piece of furniture near a wall. Place your hands on the seat,

step forward, and lower one knee, then the other, to the floor.

2. Kneeling on both knees, lower your bottom toward your heels. Use your arms and elbows, and hang on to the chair as needed. Try sitting to the sides of your feet.

3. To stand back up, reverse the process. With daily practice, your muscles will strengthen and movements will be easier.

I cannot overemphasize the importance of maintaining your ability to get up and down from the floor. It will make it easier to get up from chairs, even a toilet if the seat is low.

CHAPTER 22

YOGA DOES GET BETTER WITH AGE

The ancient yoga writings, called the *sutras*, begin with this thought: *Atha Yoga Anu Sha Sa Nam*, which means "and now we begin [the teachings]." I've long been fond of this opening because it reminds me that every day is a new beginning. Every moment, every breath, is an opportunity for a whole new start. A new beginning is always exciting! So I often begin my classes with the phrase "And now we begin."

Wisdom tells us that this moment is like no other. The poet Paul Reps (author of *Zen Flesh, Zen Bones*) reminds us, "only this moment forevers." These thoughts help me slow down and gracefully step off the train of thought that goes at breakneck speed through my day.

The future has yet to come. The joy is in the journey, not the destination. I feel like we have walked the koshas together, witness at our sides, and that you and I have become friends. New windows and doors have opened, blowing fresh air into your hatha yoga, breathing, and meditation practices. But self-reflection, with all of its benefits, comes at a price: awareness of our own mortality and vulnerability while we are alive.

The fact is I am very human. Often, with con-

cern and worry, I ask the universe, "What sort of future am I leaving to my precious grandchildren?" Soft whispers, impressions, insights quietly come. With love and respect, I'll share some with you:

Ask yourself, what would you do if everything that you hold near and dear was suddenly swept away? All that you care about, *gone*. Where would you find your heart? Where would you find your bliss?

Where? Yes, exactly . . . within the depths of your being.

All your efforts to remove the obstacles that prevent you from knowing your own bliss, truth, joy, and contentment are truly worth it.

Your efforts continue to touch all with whom

you come in contact, like ripples on a pond. First the wave washes over you. Then the ripples go out, touching your family, grandchildren, and their children and beyond, for years to come.

It takes renewed courage and patience to maintain a healthy midlife body with yin stretching, asanas, breathing, and relaxation. It takes valiant, unemotional efforts to quiet the mind through daily meditation; to think less and feel more; to make an effort to learn more from the positive emotions of joy and love, and less from fear and anger, coming to understand that every experience in our life is a teacher in disguise.

And nothing we do is a mistake. We have learned from it all. Yes, *yoga does get better with age*. Words point the way to truth, but truth cannot be contained by words.

Year after year, you and your friend the witness can do Downward-Facing Dog, and each time find something new and interesting about the pose. Again and again we can view different, subtle, deeper levels of our Self and extract what's real and meaningful, then apply it to our everyday life—remembering that if the teachings are not a part of our life, then they mean very little.

Let your apprehensions and hopes for tomorrow dissolve. No more drowning in the ouches of the past. Find joy now! Find your smile today! Reconnect with contentment now! Walk on . . . continue your midlife journey. Be the example of the changes you wish to see within family and beyond. Your inner efforts truly affect those near and dear, seen and unseen.

Perhaps one day we will meet. I'd like that very much. I send you my continued blessings, love and light upon your pathway—and know in your heart of hearts, you are not alone.

Love,

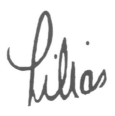

"*You cannot stay on the summit forever. You have to come down, so why bother going in the first place? JUST THIS. What is above knows what is below, but what is below does not know what is above. One climbs and one sees; one descends and one sees no longer, but one has seen. There is an art of conducting one's self in the lower region by the memory of what one saw higher up. When one no longer sees, one can at least STILL KNOW.*"

—*René Daumal*, Mount Analogue

Appendix A:
Yoga Props

Today's yoga classes use props to help stabilize poses, stretch further, and add comfort. Props can enhance your yoga practice, although it's best not to become too dependent on them. I've recommended the use of several props throughout this book.

Yoga props are easy to find and purchase at yoga studios and even many large sporting-goods stores, as well as countless Web sites. Many people, however, simply use things they already have around the house. Don't feel intimidated by props! Yoga props are here to stay and make our practice more comfortable, pleasant, and efficient.

Here are the basic props used in yoga:

YOGA MAT: Also called a "sticky mat," this is the most important prop, so if you choose to buy only one thing, this is it. A good yoga mat is slightly sticky to keep you from slipping around during practice, but most provide very little padding for your knees and back. A cheap, thin mat is almost unusable, so I don't advise selecting strictly based on price. You want your mat to be properly sticky and comfortable, yet easily portable.

I often recommend using multiple sticky mats to my students. The extra padding protects your bony knees, elbows and back and provides comfort in the poses. A three fold fitness mat is another helpful choice.

EYE PILLOWS: Placed across the eyes during relaxation, these help minimize distractions and deepen the relaxation experience. I especially enjoy an eye pillow filled with flax seeds and lavender.

BELT OR STRAP: Usually 8 feet in length, a yoga belt extends your reach, opens your shoulders and hips, and lets you increase or maintain leg and arm stretches. It usually has a side-release buckle. If you don't purchase a yoga belt, you can use a tie or sash, but be sure it's made of a sturdy enough material to support you.

BLOCKS: Blocks are used to support different parts of your body, such as hips, knees, and hands. The best blocks are light, yet sturdy and resilient, measuring about 4 inches by 6 inches by 9 inches. If you do not purchase yoga blocks, you can use large books or small boxes—just make sure whatever you choose is strong enough to support your body weight.

BLANKETS: You will need a couple of *firm* blankets. Choose one made of thick cotton or wool, such as a Mexican blanket—your grandmother's crocheted bed-throw will not work. Because blankets are used to add extra support in a posture, you don't want anything so soft that it will be flattened by your body weight. Blankets made for a twin bed work nicely. Be sure to fold them neatly and evenly to provide a smooth and level support for your body.

I often use Bheka Yoga Supplies to find quality, affordable yoga props.

Web site: www.bheka.com
Phone: 800-366-4541
E-mail: Service@bheka.com

Appendix B:
Lilias's Recommendations for Your Journey

Like most yoga teachers, I am an avid reader, and it is impossible to list all the books and articles that have influenced my view of yoga and life. The following publications were consulted during my writing of *Yoga Gets Better with Age*. Many have been quoted in the text. I'm deeply grateful to the authors of the following books and publications.

BOOKS ON YOGA

Yoga Nidra by Richard Miller - book and cd (Louisville, CO: Sounds True, Inc., 2010)

Cool Yoga Tricks by Miriam Austin (New York, NY: Ballantine Books, 2003)

Yoga at the Wall by Nancy McCaochan (Royal Oak, MI: In the Company of Women, 2008)

Beyond Power Yoga by Beryl Bender Birch (New York: Fireside, 2000).

Moving Toward Balance by Rodney Yee (Emmaus, PA: Rodale, 2004).

Yoga for Your Life by Margaret D. Pierce and Martin G. Pierce (Portland, OR: Rudra Press, 1996).

The New Yoga for People over 50 by Suza Francina (Deerfield Beach, FL: Health Communications, 1997).

Yoga for Body, Breath and Mind by A. G. Mohan (Portland, OR: Rudra Press, 1996).

The Healing Path of Yoga by Nischala Joy Devi (New York: Three Rivers Press, 2000).

Doubles Yoga, A Manual for Two or More by Shar Lee and Dawn R. Mahowald (Eastman, Quebec: Kriya Yoga Publications, 1997).

Every Woman's Yoga by Jaime Stover Schmitt (Brooklyn, NY: Prima Publishing, 2002).

Recovery Yoga by Sam Dworkis (New York: Three Rivers Press, 1997).

The Heart of Yoga by T. K. V. Desikachar (Rochester, VT: Inner Traditions, 1995).

The Now River by Nancy L. Bloemer (Now River Publications, 2003).

Yoga for Transformation by Gary Kraftsow (New York: Penguin Compass, 2002).

Relax and Renew by Judith Lasater, Ph.D., P.T. (Berkeley, CA: Rodmell Press, 1995).

Yoga for Dummies by Georg Feuerstein, Ph.D., and Larry Payne, Ph.D., foreword by Lilias Folan (Hoboken, NJ: For Dummies, 1999).

Yoga R_x by Larry Payne, Ph.D., and Richard Usatine, M.D. (New York: Broadway Books, 2002).

BOOKS FOR YOUR JOURNEY

Be Love Now by Ram Dass (New York, NY: Harper Collins, 2010)

The Possible Human by Jean Houston, Ph.D. (Kirkwood, NY: J. P. Tarcher, 1982).

The Power of Now by Eckhart Tolle (Sherman Oaks, CA: New World Library, 1999).

Agnostic Prayer by Paul Sutherland (Traverse City, MI: Karuna Press, 2004).

Yoga and the Quest for the True Self by Stephen Cope (Bantam, 2000).

Talking with Angels by Gitta Mallasz (Daimon, 2003).

BOOKS ON MEDITATION

Nine Secrets of Successful Meditation by Dr. Samprasad Vinod (London: Watkins Publishing, 2002)

Beginner's Guide to Meditation by Goswami Kriyananda (Chicago, IL: The Temple of Kriya Yoga, 2003).

Advanced Guide to Meditation by Goswami Kriyananda (Chicago, IL: The Temple of Kriya Yoga, 2003).

The Heart and Science of Yoga by Leonard Perlmutter with Jenness Cortez Perlmutter (Averill Park, NY: AMI Publishers, 2005).

BOOKS ON BREATHING

A Life Worth Breathing by Max Strom (New York, NY, Skyhorse Publishing, 2010).

The Yoga of Breath by Richard Rosen (Shambhala Publications, Inc., 2002).

BOOKS ON ANATOMY

The Endless Web by R. Louis Schultz, Ph.D., and Rosemary Feitis (North Atlantic Books, 1996).

Anatomy Trains by Thomas W. Myers (Churchill Livingstone, 2001).

Stretching and Flexibility by Kit Laughlin (Simon & Schuster Australia, 2000).

RECOMMENDED VIDEOS, CDS, AND DVDS

The Feminine Unfolding: An Exploration of Yoga with Angela Farmer (www.Angela-Victor.com).

Yoga for Scoliosis with Elise Browning Miller (www.yogaforscoliosis.com).

Yoga for Everyone with Nancy Tatum (www.Glenmoreyoga.com)

Lilias Folan DVDs and CDs and descriptions of content are available at www.liliasyoga.com.

YOGA VACATIONS WITH LILIAS

Feathered Pipe Ranch, Helena, Montana. Call (406) 442-8196 (www.Featheredpipe.com)

Kripalu, Stockbridge, MA (413) 448-3400 (www.kripalu.org)

Omega, Rhinebeck, MY (845) 266-4444 (www.eomega.org)

Yoga Journal Conferences (www.yogajournal.com)

About the Author

Master yoga teacher Lilias Folan is an American treasure known by only one name, Lilias. Since her groundbreaking 1972 PBS yoga series, *Lilias! Yoga and You*, Lilias has been described as the first "First Lady of Yoga," having spent the past three decades helping people learn about the mind, body, and spirit benefits of yoga. Regarded as America's most knowledgeable and respected master yoga teacher, Lilias has been featured on a wide selection of television shows, books, audiotapes, and videos. Her excellent reputation even prompted *Time* magazine to dub her "The Julia Child of Yoga."

Lilias first began studying yoga at the age of 30 to alleviate back problems, sleeplessness, and a general case of the "blahs." Yoga gave Lilias, then a housewife and mother, a renewed vitality and energy. With this increased zest for life, she continued her yoga practice in New York City, where she studied and taught with some of the finest teachers from Europe, India, and North America.

In 1969, Lilias began teaching classes in her Ohio community at the YWCA, sharing what she had learned. Four years later, her television series *Lilias! Yoga and You* aired on PBS stations nationwide. Today, viewers across the country continue to practice yoga with Lilias through her PBS television programs, *Lilias! III* and *Lilias! IV*, which offer a timeless, sophisticated approach to stress management and general wellness.

Lilias is featured in numerous award-winning videos, DVDs, and CDs, including:

Lilias! Alive with Yoga

Lilias! Yoga Basics

Lilias! Energize with Yoga

Lilias! Yoga for Better Health

Lilias! Flowing Posture Series

Lilias! Complete Yoga Fitness for Beginners DVD

Lilias! Yoga 101 Workout for Beginners DVD

Lilias! AM & PM Yoga Workouts for Seniors DVD

Lilias! Yoga Gets Better with Age DVD

Lilias! Yoga and You - 4 Lilias! PBS shows on 2 DVDs

The Lilias! Collection - 52 PBS shows on 16 DVDs

Discover Serenity CD

Discover Yoga - A Guided Work-in CD

The Inner Smile CD

The complete descriptions of content of the DVDs and CDs may be found at www.liliasyoga.com.

Lilias is proud to be featured in the book, *American Yoga* (Barnes & Noble), as one of 24 American master yoga teachers who have made a major contribution to yoga in America today. She is also an Advisory Council member of the *International Journal of Yoga Therapy*. In 1998, Lilias was ordained Swami Kavitananda by Goswami Kriyananda, preceptor of the Kriya Yoga Temple in Chicago. She continues to share her knowledge and experience through her global schedule of conferences, workshops, and teacher trainings. Her teaching schedule, including her YogahOMe Studio classes in Cincinnati, Ohio, may be found at www.liliasyoga.com and www.yogahome.net.

About the Photographer

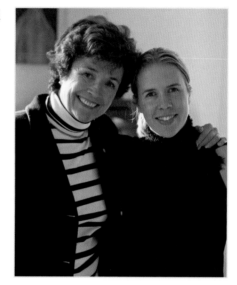

Circe Hamilton was born in 1972 and reared in London, England. She received her first camera—a Nikon, from her mother—when she was a teenager, and began snapping all of her friends. In 1991, she moved to the United States to attend Rochester Institute of Technology, from which she received her Bachelor of Fine Arts in photography. After graduation, Circe moved to New York City, where she assisted many photographers, including Vietnam War photographer Eddie Adams. Later she returned to the United Kingdom to start life as a professional photographer. Circe now lives in Gramercy, New York, but works both sides of the Atlantic. Circe's portraits can be seen in British *Elle*, British *Vogue*, and British *Esquire*, among other publications. The year 2004 marked her first solo exhibit in London at Program. This is her first book venture with her Aunt Lilias. All images were shot at the Richard Lohr studio in New York City. The shoot was playful and relaxed! Circe (www.circephoto .com) is a yoga enthusiast herself, studying at OM yoga in downtown New York.

About the Models

Nancy Glenmore Tatum, M.S., is the director of Glenmore Yoga and Wellness Center, the first yoga studio in Richmond, Virginia, which she and her husband opened in 1999. Nancy began teaching hatha yoga in 1970, with Lilias as her role model. She is certified through the Himalayan Institute and is registered as a 500-hour Senior Yoga Instructor with Yoga Alliance. Nancy has a Master of Science in gerontology and adult education and is a certified massage therapist. Nancy's video, *Yoga for Everyone*, leads beginning students through a 1-hour yoga practice. For more information on her video, e-mail Nancy at Nancy@Glenmoreyoga.com.

Kevin Patrick Casey found yoga in his twenties by way of a book by Richard Hittleman. He practiced on his own for 20 years before taking a studio class in the mid-1990s. He decided then that he was on the right path. A short time later he met his wife, Nancy, and began practicing in earnest. They married in 1997 and opened their yoga center in 1999. Kevin began teaching in 2001 and received his 200-hour certification from the Himalayan Institute the following year. He is also a certified massage therapist and incorporates assisted yoga postures as part of his approach to massage therapy.

Photo Index

A

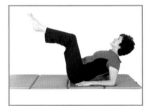

Anchored Boat Pose
(*Ardha Navasana*), 160

Bridge Pose
(*Setu Bandha*), 156

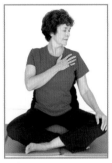

Chataranga I, 168

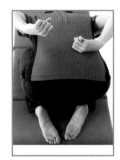

Chest Expander, Partner-
Assisted (*Yoga Mudra*),
202
Child's Pose (*Balasana*)

B

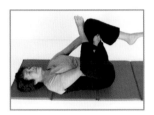

Barn Door: Piriformus
Stretch (*Supta Ardha
Padmasana*), 66

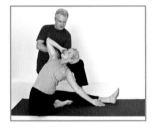

Bird of Paradise, Partner
(*Parivrtta Jan Sirsasana*),
210

C

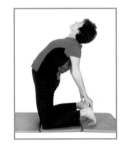

Camel, Full (*Ustrasana*),
151

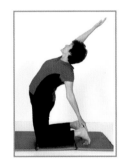

Camel, Half (*Ustrasana*),
150
Caring Breath, 130

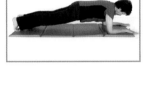

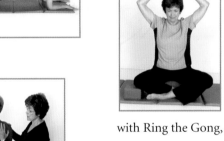

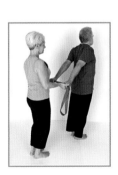

Chest Expander, 52

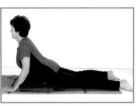

with Ring the Gong,

164
Chin to Chest, 50
Cobra Pose

(*Bhujangasana*), 162

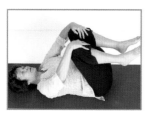

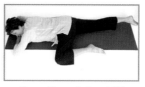

Eyes of Your Heart
Breathing, 88

F

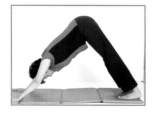

D

Dancing the Star, 113

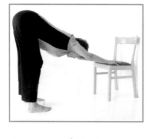

Downward-Facing Dog
(*Adho Mukha Svana-
sana*), 149
Downward-Facing Dog
with a Chair, 69

E

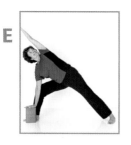

Extended Side Angle
Pose (*Utthita Parsavako-
nasana*), 184

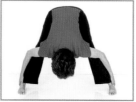

Fan Pose (*Prasarita Pa-
dottanasana*), 176

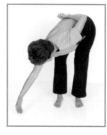

Fill the Cup, 76

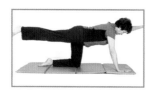

Flying Sunbird (*Chakra-
vakasana*), 144

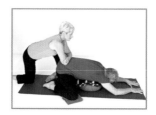

Frog Pose Solo, 115
Frog Pose, with partner

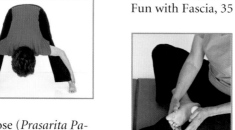

(*Bhekasana*), 212
Fun with Fascia, 35

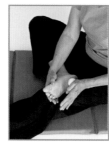

G

Garuda Arms, 57

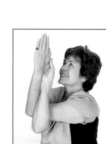

H

Half Chair Pose, 180
Half Moon Balance

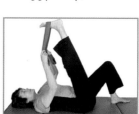

(*Ardha Chandrasana II*),

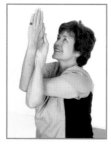

188
Hamstring Stretch,
Partner (*Supta*

Padangusthasana), 198
Hamstrings Solo, 59
Happy Baby, Partner

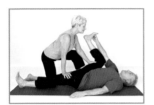

(*Supta Ekapadasana*),
213
Happy Baby with Three
Rs (*Supta Ekapadasana*),

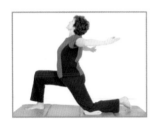

158
Heart Lunge, 132
Heart Lunge Variation,

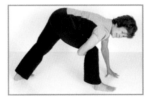

191

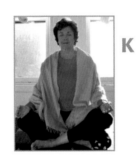

Hero's Twist (*Virasana*),

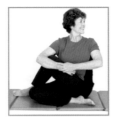

170
Hug a Tree, 68

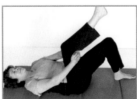

I

Inner Smile Relaxation,
128

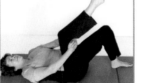

K

Knee to Chest with Three
Rs (*Vakranasana*), 64
Knees to Chest, 62

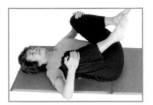

L

Legs in V Pose, 116
Legs-Up-on-the-Wall
Pose (*Viparita Karani*),
192

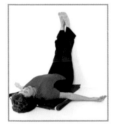

Little Mermaid Series, 72

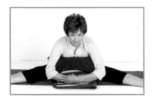

Locust Pose
(*Shalabhasana*), 165

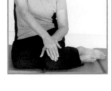

Low Back Rolling, 47

Lunge Pose (*Ashwa
Sanchalansana*), 190
Lying Down Twist, 112

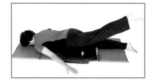

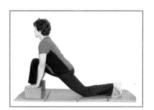

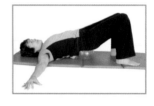

M

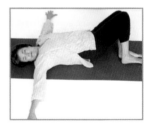

Mecca Pose, 115
Meditation, Focused, 118
Moon Breathing and

Back-to-Back Twist,
Partner, 214

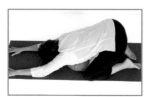

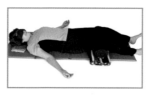

I:

Bent Knees, 146
II: Single-Leg Pigeon
Pose, 147
Piriformus with Table/

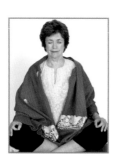

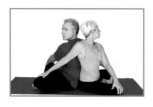

Cat/Cow, 114
Pushup (*Kapotasana*), 145

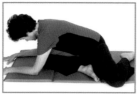

N

Neck Tilt I, 49
Neck Tilt II, 49

P

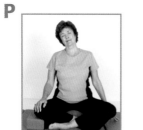

Pigeon

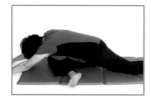

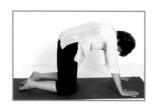

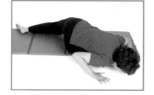

R

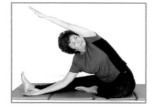

Relaxation: Sponge Pose
(*Savasana*), 195

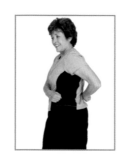

Revolving Head to Knee
(*Parivrtta Janu
Sirsasana*), 173

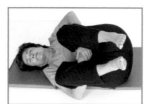

Ring the Gong, 55

Rolling Pin Series, 74

S

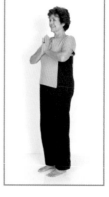

Sacred Mountain Pose
(*Tadasana*), 54

Sacred Mountain Pose
(*Tadasana*), 174

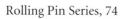

Sage Twist (*Mar-
ichyasana*), 169

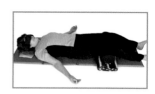

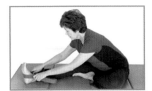

Savasana, 41
Seated Forward Bend
(*Paschimottanasana*), 172

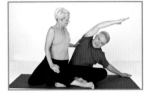

Seated Side Bend,
Partner (*Parighasana*),
207

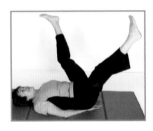

Seaweed Legs, 63

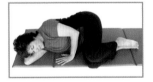

Seed Pose, 167

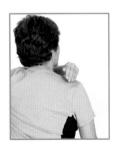

Self-Massage, 34

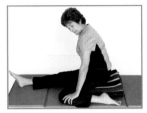

Shin Stretch with Three
Rs, 58
Shoulder Preparation for

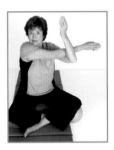

Garuda Arms, 56
Shoulder Roll, 47

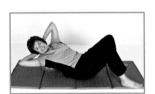

Shoulderstand, Half

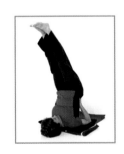

(*Salamba Sarvangasana*),
193
Side Bow Pose

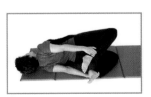

(*Dhanurasana*), 166

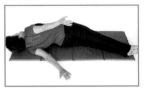

Side Cobra
(*Bhujangasana*), 166
Singing Snake, 51

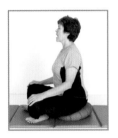

Single Leg Forward Bend,

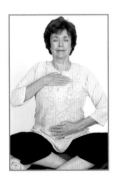

Partner (*Janu Sirsasana*),
208
Sipping Breath with

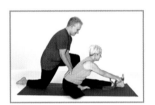

Contentment
Meditation, 119

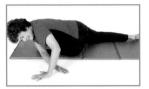

Solo Nesting Pigeon Pose
(*Kapotasana*), 148
Sphinx Pose, 161

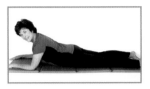

Spider on the Wall,

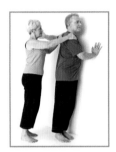

Partner, 204
Spidy on the Mat, 71

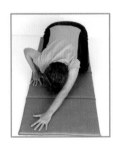

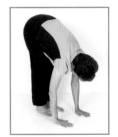

Standing Forward Bend
(*Uttanasana*), 70

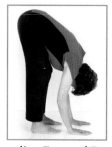

Standing Forward Bend
(*Uttanasana*), 177
Standing Forward Bend

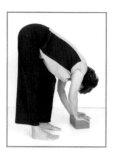

with Block (Alternating
Leg), 61
Standing Inchworm, 60

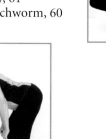

Stargazing Situp, 48

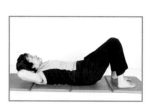

Stargazing Yogoda, 111

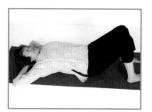

Striding Forward Bend,
178

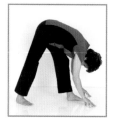

Suspension Bridge,
Partner (*Utkatasana*),

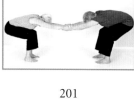

201

T

Table Pose (*Maja-*

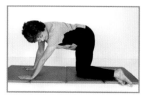

riasana) with Cat, Cow,
and Smile, 143

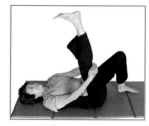

Three Rs, 44
Thunderbolt

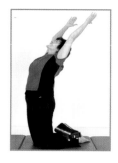

(*Vajrasana*), 152
Torso Twist I

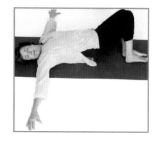

(*Parivartanasana*), 153

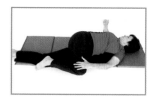

Torso Twist II
(*Jathara Parivritti*), 154

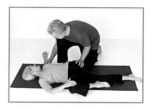

Torso Twist, Partner
(*Supta Matsyendrasana*),
200
Tree Pose, Partner

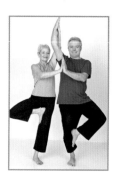

(*Vrksasana*), 206

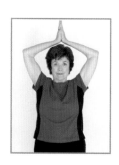

Tree Series (*Vrksasana*)
Changing Tree, 186

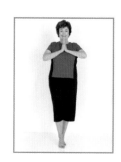

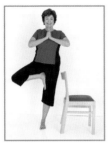

Tree, High, 186
Tree, Low, 185

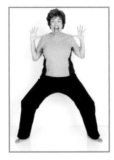
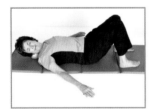

Triangle Pose (*Utthita Trikonasana*), 181

U

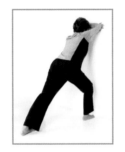

Upper Neck Curve, 46

V

W

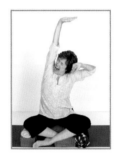

Wall Calf Stretch, 65

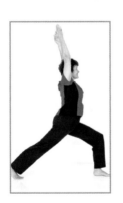

Warrior I Pose, 182

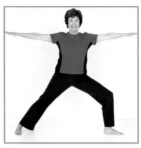

Warrior II Pose, 183

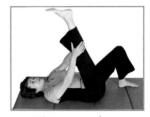

Yin approach to stretching, 43
Yoga miracle, 42

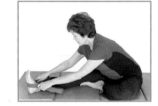

Y

Yawn with Awareness, 111

General Index

Belt(s)
    definition, 225
    for yoga, 43–45, 52, 59, 66–67, 140, 158, 168,
        173, 202, 203, 208, 213
Bhakti, xiii
Bheka Yoga Supplies, 225
Bikram yoga, 6, 9
Birch, Beryl Bender, 5
Blankets, 40, 192–94, 225
Bliss body. *See also Ananda-maya-kosha*
    connecting with, 127–29
    definition, 124–26
    introduction to, 17
Block(s)
    description of, 225
Blood pressure, 38, 39, 90, 108, 134, 193
Bone health, 10
Bramari breath, 84. *See also* Humming breath
Breath Body, 16, 80, 82, 91
Breathing, 86
Buckle up seat belt, definition, 142
Buddhist, 7
Buzz words, 142
    Buckle up seat belt, 142
    Close the gates of the shoulders, 142
    Lift the eyes of the heart, 142

C

Cancer, 100, 220
Caring Breath, 126, 130, 136, 221
Carter, President Jimmy, 80
Causal body, 15
Cave of the Heart
    definition, 109
    meditation for, 136
Challenges
    in yoga practice, 220–22
Chest
    postures for, 203
    warmups for, 52

Chidananda, Swami, 99, 125
Childbirth, 84
Choudhury, Bikram, 6
Christian, 7
Cincinnati Conservatory of Music, 125
Clean up your act, 14–15
Concentration, 5, 27. *See also* One-pointed
        attention
    improving, 21, 83, 110, 141
    introduction to, 20–21
Contentment, 24–25, 124, 136, 223–24. *See also
        Santosha*
    meditation for, 119–21
Cope, Stephen, 20
Corpse, 37, 195
Crocodile, 82, 90–91
Cushman, Anne, 94

D

Deergha Swasam, 87. *See also* Three-Part
        Breathing
Depression, 21, 97, 100, 129
Desert island, 140
Desikachar, T.K.V., 5, 6
Detach muscle, 23,
Detachment. *See also Aparigraha*
    exercise for, 23
    introduction to, 21–24
Devi, Mataji Indra, 4
Dharana. See also One-pointed
        attention
    branch of yoga, 5
    introduction to, 20–21
Dhyana
    branch of yoga, 5
    introduction to, 27
Discontent, 15, 24–25
Discover Serenity CD, 27, 29
Discover video series, 40
Donkey, stinking, 95

Douglas, Mike, 25
Dynamic movement
    definition of, 33
Dynamic tension, 38

Pain (*cont.*)
    emotional, 95–96
    naming and releasing, 98
Pain body, 96–98
Partner(s), postures for, 198–215
Patanjali, 26
Payne, Larry, 43, 118
PBS, 6, 22, 228
Perfection, 24, 125
Physical body. *See also Anna-maya-kosha*
    definition, 30–31
    introduction to, 16
Pilates, <u>41</u>
Plato, 80
PNF. *See* Proprioceptive neuromuscular
    facilitation
Postures
    choosing, 140
    five steps for, <u>141</u>
    holding, 33, 42–43, <u>141</u>
Power yoga, 5, 9
Prana, 80–81, 82
Prana-maya-kosha. See also
      Energy/breathing body
    definition, 80–81
    introduction to, 16
Pranayama
    branch of yoga, 5
    meaning of, 82
    in senior years, 11
Pranic energy, 81
Pratyahara, 26
Proprioceptive neuromuscular facilitation
    (PNF), 42
Props, 6, 140, 225
Psychotherapy, 14, 95, 97

Q

Quinn, Anthony, 25

R

Ram Dass Library, 22
Ramakrishna, Bhagavan Sri, xiii, xiv
Receiver (in partner work), 197
Relax (in three Rs), definition, 44
Relaxation, 37–41. *See also Savasana*
    deep, 39–40
    four steps of, 39–40
    introduction to, 26–27
    long exercise, 39, 40–41
    posture for, 195–96
Reps, Paul, 223
Resist, (in three Rs), definition, 44
Restlessness, 15, 16, 24, 221
Restretch, (in three Rs), definition, 44
Ripin, Crista, 66
Rishi, Bernard, xv
Rosen, Richard, 20, 84
Routines, suggested, 216–19

S

Sacred space, 108
Sakshin, 18–20, 110. *See also* Witness
Salutation to the Hips, 216
Salutation to the Moon, 218–19
Santosha, 24–25, 121. *See also* Contentment
Satsang, 24
Savasana, 37–41. *See also* Relaxation
    introduction to, 26–27
    Short Let-Go Relaxation, 37–38
    Yogoda Dynamic Relaxation, 38
Seasons, 8–11
Seated Yoga Vacation, 216
Self
    acceptance of, 15, 19
    familiarity with, 8, 16, 106
    High, 15, 16, 124
    layers of, 5, 11, 15, 17, 18, 26, 37, 124
    study of, 5, 7, 11, 25–26

Visualization. *See also* Imaging
    Cat and Mouse exercise for, 102
    definition of, 100
    exercise for, 101
    for healing, 220–21
    Train of Thought exercise for, 102
    Waterfall exercise for, 103

W

Warmup(s), 32–33, <u>32</u>, 46–77
    order of, 33
Weekend work-in, 217
Who Am I, 10, 26
Willpower, 106–7, 121
Wisdom, 8, 10, 17, 83, 106, 124, 125, 126, 220
Wisdom body. *See also Vijnana-maya-kosha*
    definition, 106–8
    development of, 121
    exercise for, 107
    introduction to, 16
    meditation for, 107–8
Witness. *See also Sakshin*
    exercise for, <u>19</u>
    introduction to, 18–20
    in meditation, 109

Witness Self. *See* Witness.
Wizard of Oz, 81
Wounds, emotional, 14, 94

Y

Yawn, anatomy of, 84–85
Yin approach
    introduction to, 42–43
    steps for, 43–44
Yin Stretches, 46–77
Yoga, definition of, 7
Yoga and the Quest for the True Self, 20
Yoga for Dummies, 43
Yoga miracle, 42–43
Yoga of Breath, The, 20
Yoga slave, 197
Yoga Sutra, 5, 26. *See also* Sutras
Yogoda Dynamic Relaxation, 38

Z

Zen Flesh, Zen Bones, 223